Cravings,
Lose
Weight!

Easy ways to let your mind do the work for you!

Warning

This book is not intended as a substitute for the attention of a medical or health practitioner. If you have symptoms for which you would normally seek assistance, you are urged to continue to do so.

The techniques described in this book are not suitable for use with helping others unless you are a fully trained health professional. To treat or guide others without sufficient training would be both irresponsible and disrespectful. Do not use these techniques with others unless you are a qualified counsellor or psychologist.

Although this book describes techniques from neuro-linguistic programming, this book is not in any way a substitute for neuro-linguistic programming training and is in no way intended to provide a discourse on, or comprehensively describe, the vast field that is neuro-linguistic programming. This book simply shows the general public how some of the more powerful techniques from both neuro-linguistic programming and neuro-somatics can be used for personal change.

Beat Cravings, Lose Weight!

Easy ways to let your mind do the work for you!

CHRISTINE SUTHERLAND

The **McGraw·Hill** Companies

Sydney New York San Francisco Auckland
Bangkok Bogotá Caracas Hong Kong
Kuala Lumpur Lisbon London Madrid
Mexico City Milan New Delhi San Juan
Seoul Singapore Taipei Toronto

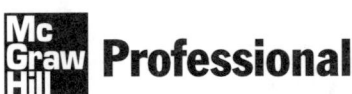 **Professional**

Text © 2004 Christine Sutherland
Illustrations and design © 2004 McGraw-Hill Australia Pty Ltd
Additional owners of copyright are named in on-page credits.

Apart from any fair dealing for the purposes of study, research, criticism or review, as permitted under the *Copyright Act*, no part may be reproduced by any process without written permission. Enquiries should be made to the publisher, marked for the attention of the Permissions Editor, at the address below.

Every effort has been made to trace and acknowledge copyright material. Should any infringement have occurred accidentally the authors and publishers tender their apologies.

Copying for educational purposes
Under the copying provisions of the *Copyright Act*, copies of parts of this book may be made by an educational institution. An agreement exists between the Copyright Agency Limited (CAL) and the relevant educational authority (Department of Education, university, TAFE, etc.) to pay a licence fee for such copying. It is not necessary to keep records of copying except where the relevant educational authority has undertaken to do so by arrangement with the Copyright Agency Limited.

For further information on the CAL licence agreements with educational institutions, contact the Copyright Agency Limited, Level 19, 157 Liverpool Street, Sydney NSW 2000. Where no such agreement exists, the copyright owner is entitled to claim payment in respect of any copies made.

Enquiries concerning copyright in McGraw-Hill publications should be directed to the Permissions Editor at the address below.

National Library of Australia Cataloguing-in-Publication data:

Sutherland, Christine, 1955– .
Beat cravings, lose weight! : easy ways to let your mind do the work for you.
Includes index.
ISBN 0 074 71384 1.
1. Weight loss — Psychological aspects. 2. Food habits. I. Title.
613.2

Published in Australia by
McGraw-Hill Australia Pty Ltd
Level 2, 82 Waterloo Road, North Ryde, NSW 2113
Acquisitions Editor: Meiling Voon
Production Editor: Rosemary McDonald
Editor: Caroline Hunter
Associate Editor: Thu Nguyen
Proofreader: Tim Learner
Indexer: Diane Harriman
Designer (cover and interior): Jan Schmoeger/Designpoint
Cover images: gettyimages
Illustrators: Lorenzo Lucia
Typeset in 12/14 pt Bembo by Jan Schmoeger/Designpoint
Printed on 80 gsm woodfree by Pantech Limited, Hong Kong.

The *McGraw·Hill* Companies

CONTENTS

	Introduction	ix
Part 1	**Finally understanding the real reasons why you are overweight**	**1**
Chapter 1	Pardon the pun, but being overweight is a big problem!	3
Chapter 2	The answer is in the brain!	9
Chapter 3	Your lousy programming	12
Chapter 4	Identifying problem behaviours: we all have our blind spots	17
Part 2	**Techniques for effortless change**	**23**
Chapter 5	The chocoholic workshop: food triggers to eating	25
Chapter 6	Excuses, excuses! Attitude to exercise	40
Chapter 7	Eating when you're not hungry: emotional triggers to eating	48
Chapter 8	The autopilot that lives your life for you: your self-image	59
Chapter 9	Thinking like a slim person	72
Chapter 10	Dealing with negative feelings: Emotional Freedom Techniques	75
Chapter 11	Internal settings: what does your unconscious mind think your ideal 'healthy' weight should be?	88

CONTENTS

Part 3	**Sabotage: how you stop yourself from getting what you want, and ways to stop the stoppers!**	**95**
Chapter 12	Identifying your sabotaging thinking and behaviour	97
Chapter 13	Using the meta model to stop criticism in its tracks: how not to get manipulated!	108
Chapter 14	Putting your weight goals to the test	120
Chapter 15	Dealing with the impact of past failures	124
Part 4	**Food and exercise**	**129**
Chapter 16	Ramping up your metabolic rate	131
Chapter 17	Food: what's normal anyway?	139
Part 5	**Planning to win**	**147**
Chapter 18	Using a weekly food plan: shave up to 75 per cent from your shopping time and family food budget!	149
Chapter 19	Your weekly exercise plan	156
Chapter 20	One step at a time: using what you've learned in an effective manner	159
Appendixes		**169**
Appendix A	Some medical reasons that may compound your weight problem: oestrogen dominance syndrome and copper toxicity	171
Appendix B	Questions/troubleshooting	174
Appendix C	What now? Support, therapy	182
Useful terms		184
Bibliography		188
Index		190

About the Author

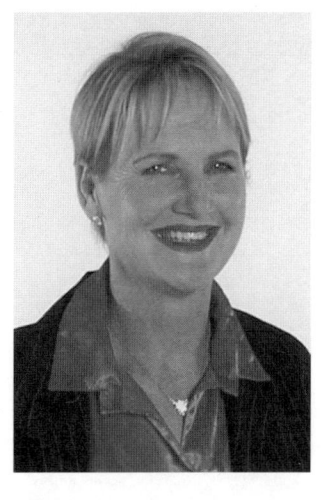

Christine Sutherland is the founding director of The Lifeworks Group, a researcher and provider of innovative mental health services, where she is responsible for clinical and training activities.

Since 1995 Christine has used her strong research and development focus to provide the most up-to-date, evidence-based applications of attitudinal and behavioural modification techniques, custom-designed for a variety of environments, from individual therapy to corporate training programs.

Christine is a consulting clinical psychotherapist with 29 years experience in counselling and training. She pioneered the introduction of neuro-somatic therapies in Australia, and is an advanced trainer in Emotional Freedom Techniques, as well as Be Set Free Fast, having been trained by the developer of the method, Dr Larry Phillip Nims. She is registered with the Australian Counselling Association as a clinical supervisor.

Christine has been responsible for the development of an innovative group treatment program for clinical depression, subjected to experimental trial in December 2000; the 'Get a Life!' program for schools, subjected to experimental trial in April/May 2000; 'PhysEd', a new approach to the treatment of chronic unresolved physical pain, subjected to clinical trial in January 2002; and, most recently, the

ABOUT THE AUTHOR

completion of a radical program to achieve permanent weight control. She has treated over 1800 clients.

Christine is married to John Sutherland and has two children, two stepchildren and a dog called Tarzan. She is an enthusiastic tennis player who unashamedly uses her knowledge of neuro-linguistic programming and neuro-somatics to improve her performance on the court. Her motto is: 'This stuff is just too good to use only for clients!'

Introduction

We have always known deep down that diets don't provide lifelong change. Yet never before have so many diets, pills and programs been available. Are they helping? No way! Not only is the obesity rate increasing dramatically in every Western country, but we're also seeing shocking obesity rates in our children.

Every year, millions of dieters put on so much weight that they end up heavier than when they started. In addition, many children who start on diets find that they cannot stop and develop problems such as anorexia or bulimia.

Our diet-obsessed society is in fact *creating* obesity and eating disorders!

So, where are you right now?

Hopefully, you've fully realised that fad or deprivation dieting is never going to get you the permanent results that you want and so you are at least willing to look at a genuine breakthrough that can have you throwing away the kilojoule/calorie counters, scales, tape measure and fat pills—*permanently*. Your reward will be a life where you can feel totally free around food—a life of fun, health and vitality.

How? By relieving yourself of the burden of the lousy programming that has had you making poor choices around food and exercise. Think about it. When you were born, there was no way you could possibly eat more food than you needed. You actually had to be taught to do this. Similarly, when you were little, there was no way anyone could keep you still. You had to learn to do this too. Luckily, that original programming, where stuffing yourself is unthinkable and avoiding opportunities to 'play' is equally unlikely, is still there and ready to come to the fore.

How do I know? Because I've done it myself and used it with hundreds of clients. What I absolutely know for sure is that when people use these simple techniques, they work!

Are there any failures? You bet! If you simply read this book and then put it away in a drawer without using it, you will fail for sure. If you use it just a bit and avoid opportunities for change, you will also fail. I haven't worked out a way to force people to use this knowledge and I've got no intention of doing so. I can only tell you that if you keep doing what you've always done, you'll keep getting what you've always got. If that's what you genuinely want, be my guest and pass on this book to someone who'll actually use it. On the other hand, if you genuinely want to be slimmer and healthier, this book can tell you how.

What techniques are used in this book?

Health experts around the world are now joining me in saying that willpower and positive thinking alone are not the answer to weight problems. The addictive/compulsive components of any weight problem, and the emotional factors that underlie weight problems, are just not amenable to willpower.

Sure, we can stick to our diet or whatever for a little while (maybe), but inevitably we crack and it all goes to hell in a hand basket. There we are, right back where we started—or even worse.

So, the techniques described in this book have very little to do with using willpower to control eating. I'd have to be insane to suggest an approach that's been failing for decades! Instead, the techniques used are the latest behavioural modification tools—tools that are aimed not at your conscious will, but at your unconscious mind.

You see, it's not your conscious mind that produces the cravings. If it were, you could switch it off any time you wanted! Truly, it's your unconscious mind that produces these cravings, against your will! It's your unconscious mind you must make an impact on.

NEURO-LINGUISTICS AND NEURO-SOMATICS

'Neuro-linguistics' and 'neuro-somatics' are words you won't hear often in most psychologists' offices. Although the approaches are 30 years old and 10 years old, respectively, nothing changes quickly in the field of health care and it'll probably be another 30 years before most health practitioners catch up!

How do I know these approaches work? Well, I certainly wouldn't just 'try them out' on you! I've been using these techniques therapeutically with individuals and groups for most of the last decade. Over the last three years The Lifeworks Group has put these techniques to clinical trial in three different clinical research projects, one of which has been peer-reviewed and published in the academic journal *Frontier Perspectives*. The group's research papers are on the web site *www.lifeworks-group.com.au* for you to see for yourself.

The results The Lifeworks Group has achieved using these techniques are nothing short of spectacular. Literally, such results have never been achieved before in the history of behavioural science. So it's no wonder I am so confident, is it?

Some of you reading this book may have been exposed to some of these techniques before. You may have heard of NLP (neuro-linguistic programming), BSFF (Be Set Free Fast) and EFT (Emotional Freedom Techniques). However, you don't need to understand these techniques to make use of this book.

- *NLP* is an incredibly broad and deep field, and is sometimes called the 'science of subjective perception'. It was developed by Richard Bandler (a mathematician) and John Grinder (a linguist) and is based on observation and analysis of excellence in communication and behaviour. It has incredible implications for sport, psychology, business and just about any other sector you can think of. A knowledge of NLP allows you to alter your automatic thinking or behaviour so that, rather than merely 'trying' to think or behave in a different way, the change is effortless (there is no 'trying'). For example, you may have a behaviour that involves feeling bored, going to the pantry and finding something to eat, even though you're not hungry. Using an NLP technique called the resource triangle, you can break this pattern permanently in just a few minutes. You no longer have to use willpower to keep yourself

INTRODUCTION

out of the pantry. In fact, you will tend to forget about the pantry altogether!

- *BSFF* is a technique not a field. Originally, BSFF relied on tapping acupoints in combination with instructions to the subconscious. More recently, its developer, American clinical psychologist Dr Larry Phillip Nims, removed this factor (a hangover from its kinesiological roots) and, lo and behold, the technique still worked. BSFF seems especially useful in addressing the self-esteem or trauma issues that might underpin some overeating behaviours.
- *EFT* is also a technique not a field and was developed about the same time as BSFF. EFT is still the 'tapping' technique that American Gary Craig originally developed, but it has gone through several modifications. The insistence that EFT works by impacting on the body's 'energy' system is highly questionable, verging on the nonsensical, but this should not distract us from the fact that it has an effect that is both significant and reliable. EFT shines when it comes to quickly and permanently eliminating negative emotional reactions. For example, you might feel deprived at the thought of going without a second helping. That feeling of deprivation can be eliminated very quickly indeed with EFT.

There is no such thing as a technique that works for all people 100 per cent of the time. Also, depending on the problem, some techniques are more easily applied than others. Therefore, it makes sense to have at your fingertips a range of the most powerful techniques for permanent change known to modern science. Because of the overlaps between NLP, BSFF and EFT, you can mix and match, and even use them simultaneously as you become more skilled and creative.

How to use this book

The first thing I recommend is that you read this book thoroughly and thoughtfully without necessarily trying anything out. But, as I said at the start, if you just read the book and don't actually use it, nothing will change! To get results, you must *apply what you learn*, and the best way to do this is through a plan.

For this reason, at the back of the book you'll find an exercise planner (see Chapter 19), a food planner (see Chapter 18) and a 12-week program (see Chapter 20). Together these will help you to get into a

INTRODUCTION

healthy routine. The food planner will not only help you with a routine, it might also save you hours of shopping time and perhaps many hundreds of dollars!

If you have health problems that require a specialised diet, do not alter your eating plan without consulting your medical practitioner, dietician or nutritionist. If you have been inactive, do not take up an exercise plan without checking with your medical practitioner.

In the 12-week program, you'll find instructions for targeting problems such as cravings. In these instructions, you'll be directed to the part of the book that teaches the technique(s) required.

Some people prefer to make up their own plans and strategies, which is wonderful. However, others gain confidence from having things set out for them. Either way is fine. The important thing is that you *do it*.

I hope you enjoy this book and find it useful.

Part 1
Finally understanding the real reasons why you are overweight

Chapter 1
Pardon the pun, but being overweight is a big problem!

WEIGHT-RELATED PROBLEMS are the leading cause of disease in the developed world. Our hospitals are clogged with patients who are suffering from the many complications of obesity and our health system is on the brink of collapse. As a society we desperately need to step off the diet merry-go-round and say goodbye to diets, pills, potions and shakes. When we do this by changing our unconscious programming, we move effortlessly and naturally towards the best health that we can have, simultaneously helping our wallets, our families and our health system.

This chapter will help you to:
- ✓ Recognise why even the healthiest diets can't help the 60 per cent of Australians who are overweight.
- ✓ Learn that dieting is a deadly trap that actually damages your health and wellbeing.
- ✓ Understand that dieting is also a deadly trap because it sets your focus on food instead of physical activity!
- ✓ Realise that if you're doing it tough, you're doing it wrong!

PART 1 UNDERSTANDING WHY YOU ARE OVERWEIGHT

In Australia, the latest National Nutrition Survey shows that 45 per cent of women and 65 per cent of men are overweight. Over the last 20 years our obesity rate has doubled to 17 per cent of men and 19 per cent of women. According to the National Health and Medical Research Council's paper *Acting on Australia's Weight*, our children are two to three times more likely to be obese as children's obesity rates have trebled in the last decade!

The costs of being overweight are enormous: every year, over $700 million is spent from the public purse and over $500 million is spent by individuals attending diet or weight-loss clinics. Our hospitals are full of people who have diseases that are a direct consequence of being overweight, such as heart disease, metabolic disorders, diabetes, oedema, osteoarthritis, gallbladder disease, cancer of the endometrium, biliary system disease and respiratory problems. The costs in loss of life are even worse. Every year in Australia we lose many thousands of people to the effects of being overweight. We also lose *thousands* of young women every year as a result of dieting diseases such as anorexia and bulimia. I hate to think how many more thousands are lost in countries with higher populations.

So, what's wrong with dieting? Isn't it better to keep dieting than to just let yourself get fatter? If being overweight is killing us, surely it's better to try to diet and lose that weight? When you look at the damage that diets do, you begin to see that not only do diets *not* lead to an overall weight loss, they actually lead to more weight gain!

Look at the diet merry-go-round in Figure 1.1. Is this the pattern of your life, as it has been for millions of others?

Who hasn't experienced this pattern, over and over again? Rather than deciding to lose weight for health reasons, most of us get to this point because we are unhappy with our appearance, or because we feel fat or unattractive. That's when you get on the diet merry-go-round:

1. You decide to go on yet another diet, setting food rules and denying yourself certain foods that you've previously enjoyed. You go without from sheer willpower.
2. Naturally, you experience feelings of deprivation, not just physical but also emotional, and this leads to much frustration as you continue to try to force yourself to live by the diet rules.
3. Sooner or later you feel angry and resentful. You may have lost weight in the beginning and now, not realising that you've affected

CHAPTER 1 BEING OVERWEIGHT IS A BIG PROBLEM!

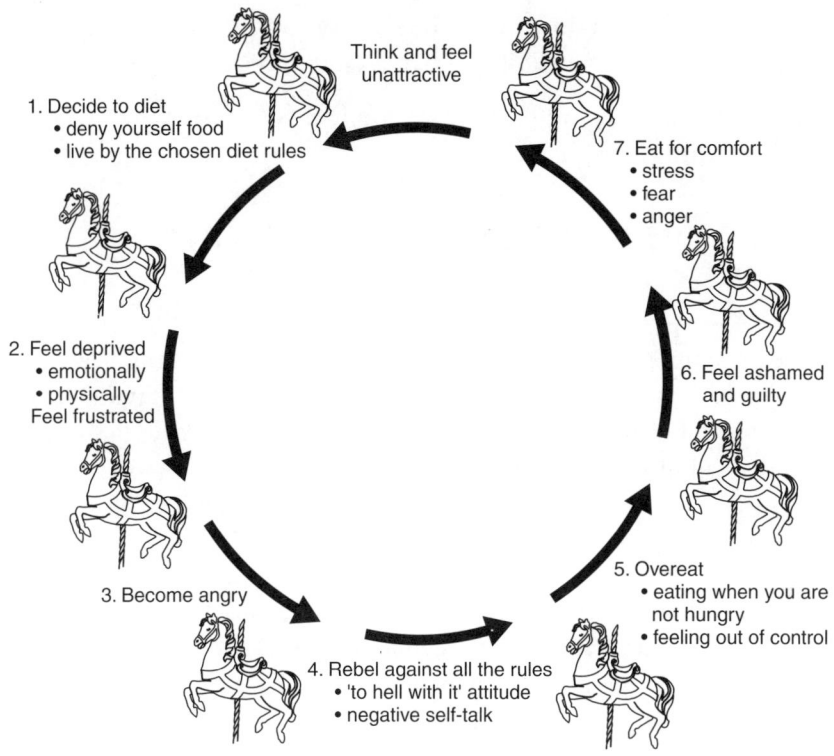

Figure 1.1 The diet merry-go-round

your metabolic rate, you can't understand why it's not shifting any more. Your mood goes up with weight loss and plummets down when the loss doesn't continue. People around you find you hard to live with.

4. The anger and resentment build into a sort of crescendo until you explode in rebellion. To hell with it!
5. As you blast out of your diet, you eat anything and everything—it's all or nothing at this point. Either you're on the diet or you'll eat that whole packet of biscuits! There's no in-between! Often at this stage the eating is sneaky—behind the pantry door, because you feel embarrassed that you can't 'stick' to the diet. You hate yourself because you're totally out of control and powerless to do anything about it.
6. Now you feel really bad—upset, disappointed, angry, guilty and ashamed.

PART 1 UNDERSTANDING WHY YOU ARE OVERWEIGHT

7. And what do you do when you feel bad? Comfort eat! Yes, you eat and eat until the turmoil and bad feelings are over, but then ...

You look at yourself and realise that you feel fat or unattractive ... and the whole thing starts again!

Why you couldn't lose weight, even on a diet

For years many people on diets have been frustrated because they have failed to lose weight, or have even gained it, despite having strictly adhered to their diet program. Nutritional research throws light on the physiology behind this distressing experience. Dr David Watts, a nutritional researcher, discusses the neurological effects of kilojoule (calorie) restriction on weight control:

> The autonomic nervous system, consisting of the sympathetic and parasympathetic branches, has a significant influence on the metabolic rate. The sympathetic branch has a stimulating effect and the parasympathetic branch a sedative effect. Evidence shows that dominance of either branch will affect body fat distribution. It is interesting to note that fasting and caloric restriction suppresses the sympathetic or stimulatory branch, thus antagonising weight loss in the majority of individuals (Watts 1993).

So, fasting and kilojoule restriction actually lower your metabolism. In fact, your body interprets fasting and kilojoule restriction as an attack on your wellbeing—posing a dangerous risk of starvation—and lowers your metabolic rate in order to ensure your survival.

But that's not all. When your metabolic rate lowers, you also experience less energy and less interest in life, and become less active. Typically, your libido also suffers. Often, you struggle to think straight or make sound decisions. You become more fatigued but paradoxically seem unable to gain refreshment from sleep. Your lower metabolism affects other body and brain functions and detracts from your quality of life!

Let me demonstrate how your body responds to just *thinking about* kilojoule restriction. I've made it fairly extreme so that the effects are obvious.

CHAPTER 1 BEING OVERWEIGHT IS A BIG PROBLEM!

EXERCISE

Imagine that, from this very moment on, I am putting you on a kilojoule-restricted diet. Your meals for the next four weeks will consist of a rice cracker, a lettuce leaf, some boiled egg white and half a tomato. When the hunger pangs grip, you can drink only water.

As you imagined this, were you aware of a sensation perhaps in your gut or your chest area that felt like a contraction or tension? This is your body reacting quite instinctively and unconsciously to the thoughts you were having about kilojoule restriction. The diet wasn't even real—you were just cooperating with me and imagining it, but it had an effect anyway!

So, not only does weight-loss dieting lower your metabolism, but even *thinking* about fasting or food restriction can have the same effect. No wonder people put on so much weight when they come off their diets!

Now, if diets were merely useless, perhaps they wouldn't be so bad after all. But, as you can see from the list below, diets are far worse than merely useless! The following list of diet problems is compiled from research around the world.

1. With weight-loss dieting, what is often lost is not fat, but fluid and muscle mass, further compromising your metabolic rate and your health. Fluid in particular can be stripped off very fast, but of course it returns amazingly quickly as well! It is physically impossible for most people to eliminate more than 0.5–1 kg per week in actual fat. If you're losing more than that, you're probably lowering your metabolism through fluid or muscle loss.
2. Diets have been linked with eating disorders, particularly among children and children of mothers who have dieted.
3. Weight-loss dieting can cause health problems and can even lead to gall bladder disease if the weight loss is too rapid.
4. Weight-loss dieting is strongly linked to a lowered metabolic rate. The reason that many older women have difficulty losing weight is not their age! They have literally stuffed up their metabolism! (Luckily, this can be rectified.)
5. Dieting has been linked with a lowered libido. Diets can wreck a great sex life!

PART 1 UNDERSTANDING WHY YOU ARE OVERWEIGHT

6. Diets usually cost money, money that could have been spent on lovely new clothes or family treats. If diets worked, this would be a wise investment. The problem is, the effects are merely temporary!
7. Diets often don't provide correct nutrition, leading to problems with concentration and memory and also to decreased wellbeing.
8. Food deprivation causes food cravings!

So why diet? The effect is temporary at best, and it causes serious problems for your health and wellbeing.

Should you just decide to stay fat? With 20 per cent of hospital deaths directly related to being overweight, I don't believe this is an option! The 'Big is Beautiful' brigade have a lot to answer for! There is no reason for us to tolerate the problems of overweight and obesity in our community, especially now that there *is* an answer! To understand that answer you first need to understand the *real* reasons for weight gain. Read Chapter 2 to find out all about it!

Note

This permanent approach to weight loss requires no 'willpower towards food' whatsoever. If you are 'trying' to lose weight, depriving yourself of foods you enjoy, talking yourself out of having what you want or forcing yourself to suffer through exercise you don't enjoy, you are not only doing it wrong, you are wasting opportunities to normalise your weight automatically and permanently. If you are doing it tough, you are doing it wrong!

CHAPTER 2
The answer is in the brain!

YOUR CONSCIOUS MIND absolutely does not 'run the show'. No matter what you want consciously, it is your unconscious mind and its automatic, conditioned responses that control your thoughts, your behaviours and your choices.

This chapter will help you to:

✓ Understand why your food and lifestyle preferences are not under your conscious control, but are merely conditioned responses, or unconscious learnings.

✓ Realise that if you want to create change in your life, you must change your unconscious mind, not your conscious mind.

✓ Learn about NLP techniques—the tools that allow you to change your preferences at the deepest level possible, your unconscious mind, putting yourself on autopilot to a healthier, happier life.

PART 1 UNDERSTANDING WHY YOU ARE OVERWEIGHT

Information from every single event in your life enters the brain through an organ called the thalamus. This organ can be thought of as the gatekeeper of the brain. From there, the information is 'coded' for emotional meaning by the hippocampus and the amygdala. These emotionally loaded 'meanings' then arrive at the frontal cortex, where they dominate any decision you attempt to make, including decisions about things as basic as eating, drinking and moving our bodies.

Figure 2.1 shows the location of the thalamus, hippocampus and amygdala in the brain, the parts of the brain primarily responsible for the formation of conditioned responses. Emotionally loaded information from the hippocampus and amygdala floods the frontal cortex whenever you try to assess, judge or make a decision about anything. No wonder it's almost impossible to choose 100 per cent rationally!

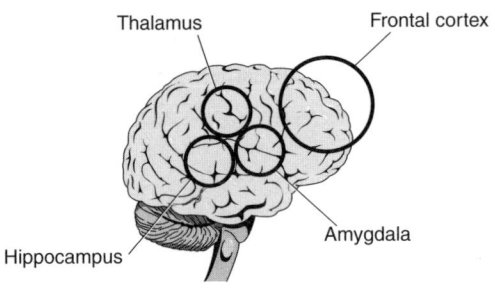

Figure 2.1 How the brain generates emotional responses

The hippocampus and amygdala together are responsible for memory, learning and emotion. They are very much interdependent and are the basis of conditioned, automatic learning. In other words, this mechanism produces automatic associations between stimuli (events) and responses (automatic feelings or behaviours). This is why people respond to certain music, smells, faces or maybe foods!

The whole stimulus–response process happens faster than the conscious mind can possibly track (see Figure 2.2). On receiving a stimulus, the brain reacts within 0.02 seconds. This is the reason it has been so difficult to make the best choices for your body. Unconsciously, the choice has already been made. Presented with information, the unconscious mind selects its choice nearly half a second before you become aware you even have a choice!

CHAPTER 2 THE ANSWER IS IN THE BRAIN!

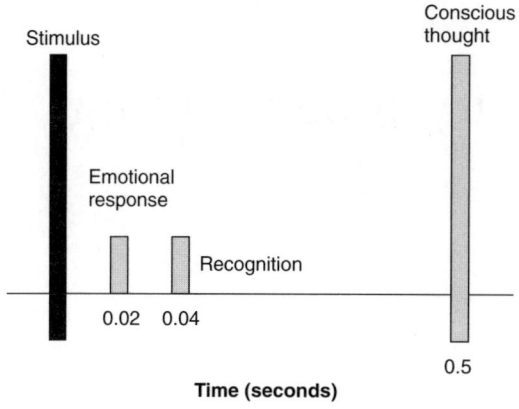

Figure 2.2 Timeline showing how unconscious processing precedes conscious thought

Hypnotherapy has recognised this but has attempted to deal with the problem simplistically by merely giving hypnotic commands. These are mostly doomed to failure over time as the automatic 'failsafe' system that was part of the original programming senses the incongruity of commands that mismatch programming and pulls our whole system, body and mind, back into line—back into old, unhelpful habits.

NLP techniques can be used to work on your unconscious programming and choices, making change effortless, natural and permanent. And NLP techniques not only attend to your basic programming, but also to the automatic 'failsafes' that have in the past sabotaged your efforts over time. With this approach, if you're trying, you are definitely doing it wrong! Willpower is not allowed!

CHAPTER 3
Your lousy programming

THE ANSWER TO WEIGHT PROBLEMS is not going on a diet or suffering through exercise. Rather, it lies in accessing and modifying the unconscious programming that automatically controls your diet and exercise preferences. This chapter looks at just some of the programming 'glitches' that NLP techniques can treat—easily, rapidly and permanently.

This chapter will help you to:

✓ Understand the complex 'ecology' of programming that controls your individual likes and dislikes.

✓ Realise that, thanks to advances like NLP, BSFF and EFT, this whole ecology is amenable to permanent change.

CHAPTER 3 YOUR LOUSY PROGRAMMING

The NLP approach to weight problems works because it fully appreciates and addresses the complexity of issues that underpin weight disorders (both overweight and underweight). Many of these issues are common in people generally, and some are quite unique to the individual and must be discovered and treated. This is not a 'by the numbers' or 'recipe' style of approach.

When you see just some of the issues that impact on body weight, you will begin to understand not only the complexity of the problem, but also why the results that The Lifeworks Group has achieved have been so easy and so outstanding. Keep in mind as you review the list below that until now most of these issues were either untreatable or were treatable only after many years of intensive therapy. Clinical research done right here in Australia proves the rapid effectiveness of The Lifeworks Group's methods in eliminating every single block to choosing your best weight.

- nutrition behaviour
- lifestyle behaviour
- eating strategies
- family history, beliefs, values
- addictive/compulsive components
- appetite
- feelings about food and weight
- feelings about sexuality/gender
- feelings about relationships
- advantages of excess weight
- disadvantages of excess weight
- disadvantages of losing weight
- advantages of losing weight
- fantastical thinking
- identity issues
- esteem/confidence issues
- unconscious programming around weight, including your internal 'setting'!

It is no wonder that diets don't work! How could they when they don't even begin to attend to the real causes of weight disturbance? How could they when diet consultants have no or little understanding of the way unconscious programming works, or of how this programming may be very readily altered?

PART 1 UNDERSTANDING WHY YOU ARE OVERWEIGHT

What we all learned growing up

- *Finish what's on your plate or you won't get your pudding!*
- *You can't leave the table until you finish your plate!*
- *Finish your plate—there are children starving in Africa!*
- *Your mother cooked that and you'll eat it!*

Who hasn't grown up hearing these comments at least a million times? No wonder it's almost impossible for a grown adult to push away a plate of food without feeling some guilt. And if you were one of several children, at meal times did you have to get in quickly before the others got everything? Did your parents use food to reward you, to quieten you, to console you or to shut you up? Guess what? You learned the 'meaning' of food and chances are you're still living that out today.

There are thousands of pieces of programming inside your head that run automatically. Collectively, these form the autopilot that runs your life when you're not looking. Like any autopilot, it follows a set of rules, or programming, that respond to feedback in order to stay on its designated track. If the programming contains an error, the autopilot won't recognise the error—it will just keep on flying right into the mountain or storm, because it doesn't think for itself.

Your lifestyle choices: do you think you decide using your own free will? Think again!

What is it that causes you to make the same unhealthy choices about food and physical exercise over and over again? Are you actually making such decisions from your own free will? Do you sabotage yourself deliberately? What is going on?

All of us engage in repetitive habits that have built up over a lifetime, and anyone who's ever tried to deliberately change a habit will know what a hard job it is to try to do it by willpower. Talk about frustrating!

However, once you understand some simple facts about neurology, you'll realise that it's not about willpower—it's about unconscious conditioning!

What do I mean by 'unconscious conditioning'? Have you heard of Pavlov and his dogs? Pavlov was a behavioural scientist who was

CHAPTER 3 YOUR LOUSY PROGRAMMING

very interested in how animals (including humans) learned to behave in automatic ways. He ran a famous experiment on dogs whereby every time the dogs were fed, a tuning tine would be rung. He soon discovered that if the tuning tine were rung, even with no food, the dogs would increase their salivation rates. They had learned to associate the sound with food, and their brains had linked a stimulus (the sound) with a response (salivation).

We humans have many, many stimulus-response associations. When we hear a special song, we feel a special way. When we see someone's hand reaching towards us in handshake, we find our own hand rising by itself. When we smell onions sizzling on a barbecue, our mouths water even though we're not hungry. When we attempt to leave a half-full plate on the table, we get the same guilty feeling we got as a child with the old 'There are children starving in Africa' routine from Mum or Dad. Certain sights, sounds, touches, smells and tastes cause us to feel or behave in very predictable ways.

Now you might be thinking, 'I can be aware of that and stop it'. The trouble is, there's too much to be aware of. Your unconscious mind is running several million responses at any given time. Your conscious mind can track only about seven of them over the same period. That's a pretty big gap! In addition, your unconscious mind responds before you even consciously become aware of it. How do you 'stop' something that's already happened?

When you realise how the mind and body work together, this strange problem becomes quite easy to understand. Simply put, it is not your conscious mind that runs your life at all. We are operating under a total misconception if we think that we are 'in control'. We are not. Our unconscious mind makes decisions even before our conscious mind realises that a decision can be made.

Our unconscious mind responds automatically and rapidly (in less than 0.02 seconds) to stimuli like food. Our unconscious mind presents us with all our attitudes and feelings about food and exercise, and our conscious mind is merely the recipient!

This is exactly why it is not your fault if you are overweight. There is literally nothing you can consciously do about it. You are like the 'ex' smoker who becomes aware that they are standing at the cigarette counter taking change for a packet of cigarettes they don't even remember asking for. The unconscious mind will have its way!

PART 1 UNDERSTANDING WHY YOU ARE OVERWEIGHT

Now this might sound pretty depressing, but in fact it's quite the opposite! Now that you properly appreciate and understand the true nature of the problem, you can stop wasting your time trying to apply willpower and actually do something different. If you want a different result, use a different strategy!

Fortunately, there is something that can unconsciously be done about this serious problem. Using techniques from NLP, BSFF and EFT, you can extinguish (eliminate) all conditioned responses around food so that you revert to your original, healthy programming. This is the key to permanent change.

Chapter 4
Identifying problem behaviours: we all have our blind spots

MOST OVERWEIGHT PEOPLE have unhealthy behaviour that they may not even be aware of until someone brings it to their attention. Even then, there may be some denial of the behaviour actually being a 'problem'.

This chapter will help you to:
- ✓ Discover whether you are under the control of food.
- ✓ Realise that there may be emotional reasons for your poor eating choices.
- ✓ Recognise poor eating behaviour.
- ✓ Recognise problem areas relating to exercise.
- ✓ Recognise how you may be sabotaging your metabolic rate.

PART 1 UNDERSTANDING WHY YOU ARE OVERWEIGHT

FOOD BEHAVIOURS AND EMOTIONS THAT NEED HELP

A word about pigging out! Pigging out, binging, feasting and eating just for the heck of it because it's a special occasion are all perfectly normal, enjoyable, healthy human activities. Doing this once every few months makes no difference whatsoever to your weight. A problem only arises when this becomes commonplace in your life. If this happens, you need to admit that you are out of control because this is absolutely not healthy or normal human behaviour.

Here are some examples of behaviour that certainly is a problem if it occurs regularly:

- ❏ snacking on biscuits or confectionery
- ❏ being out of control with certain foods
- ❏ knowing certain foods are your 'weakness'
- ❏ deliberately not buying certain foods because you know you'll eat them all
- ❏ going back to that cake/treat in the refrigerator again and again … until it's all gone
- ❏ making excuses to 'reward' yourself with food that you know isn't good for you
- ❏ hiding treats around the house because you feel guilty about eating them
- ❏ eating in secret
- ❏ stealing your children's lollies or treats
- ❏ being unable to stop once you start eating
- ❏ eating to fill a 'void' rather than for hunger
- ❏ eating for emotional reasons like stress, or boredom, or loneliness
- ❏ regularly eating in the car or in front of the television
- ❏ obsessively thinking about food all through the day—it's almost always on your mind
- ❏ feeling you can't get by without it
- ❏ fearing 'missing out', so you put more than you really need on your plate
- ❏ feeling guilty over wasting food

CHAPTER 4 IDENTIFYING PROBLEM BEHAVIOURS

- ❏ feeling resentment over 'having' to eat healthy food
- ❏ drinking carbonated beverages instead of water
- ❏ drinking more than two cups/glasses of caffeinated beverage or alcohol per day
- ❏ eating high-energy foods inappropriately (e.g. a large handful of nuts is equivalent to an extra meal)
- ❏ eating fatty or rich foods (e.g. desserts, junk food, Chinese takeaway, fried or crumbed foods, sauces)
- ❏ thinking about food throughout the day
- ❏ feeling 'needy' about food
- ❏ fearing starvation or deprivation
- ❏ avoiding salads
- ❏ craving food of any kind
- ❏ going back for seconds
- ❏ (if you are a woman) eating the same portions as your male partner
- ❏ feeling anger or sadness about making changes
- ❏ eating for social reasons
- ❏ eating when not hungry
- ❏ feeling dislike or disgust for food you know is good for you
- ❏ feeling resentful of others eating
- ❏ feeling that you should 'finish your plate'
- ❏ accepting food you do not want
- ❏ vomiting or wishing to vomit after eating
- ❏ making up excuses to eat
- ❏ not wanting to treat something because it is scary or upsetting to think about not having the problem any more (e.g. loving pizza and being afraid of what it would be like not to love pizza).

If you are engaged in any of these behaviours, then you are certainly under the control of your food! Of course, you can stay that way if you wish, but then you also get to keep your weight problem.

Are you feeling scared? Are you concerned about 'going without' or 'missing out'? Be very careful here. I am not telling you to stop. *I am not telling you to stop.* I am telling you to eat whatever you want, whenever you want. By treating your food triggers successfully, you'll never need to use willpower again. You'll never feel fearful about food again.

PART 1 UNDERSTANDING WHY YOU ARE OVERWEIGHT

Exercise behaviours and emotions that need help

Once upon a time we didn't call it exercise, we called it 'play'. When you were small and caught up in some great 'game', hot, red and sweaty with your hair plastered to your head and a big grin on your face, and Mum called you to dinner, were you interested? No way!

Just because you're grown-up now, doesn't mean you've lost your right to play! What's getting in the way of your loving the feeling of moving your body? What's getting in the way of your getting your life back again and getting out there and playing for the fun of it?

Here are some examples of unhelpful attitudes, beliefs and behaviours around physical activity:

- ❏ hating exercise of any kind
- ❏ feeling low in energy
- ❏ believing that there is simply not the time to exercise
- ❏ believing that some people (you) just aren't suitable for exercise or don't really need it
- ❏ thinking that slow walking is adequate for health
- ❏ thinking that gardening or housework is enough
- ❏ thinking that watching someone else exercise is enough!
- ❏ feeling embarrassed about exercising in front of people
- ❏ thinking that you may eat more because you've exercised
- ❏ thinking that coasting downhill on a bicycle is exercise
- ❏ thinking if you watch an exercise video it 'rubs off'
- ❏ having excuses not to exercise: too tired, too early, too late, too cold, too hot, too …
- ❏ having fears about exercise that are not backed up by your medical practitioner
- ❏ fearing the normal 'good' ache of a muscle that's been well worked
- ❏ feeling self-blame, disappointment, hopelessness, guilt, struggle, etc.
- ❏ feeling like you 'deserve' a break from exercise
- ❏ thinking of exercise as a punishment or struggle
- ❏ feeling dislike or disgust for exercise
- ❏ feeling resentful about exercise

CHAPTER 4 IDENTIFYING PROBLEM BEHAVIOURS

- feeling that you shouldn't have to exercise
- feeling fat or ugly, or indeed having any negative feelings about your body in movement.

BEHAVIOURS AND THOUGHTS THAT WORK AGAINST YOUR METABOLIC RATE

Your metabolic rate is indeed your 'life force'. If your metabolic rate is low, not only will you find it difficult to lose weight, but you also will probably battle with fatigue and depression.

Did you know that 70 per cent of the energy you burn every day is burned by your *resting* metabolic rate? That means sleeping, sitting down and standing still use up 70 per cent of your daily energy requirements. This means that your resting metabolic rate is the most important single factor that impacts on your weight.

There is an enormous amount that you can do to increase your metabolic rate, which, by the way, automatically increases your sense of wellbeing and energy. But first, you need to understand what you've been doing to sabotage your metabolic rate!

Here are some examples of beliefs, attitudes and behaviours that sabotage your metabolism:

- following a cycle of dieting, losing weight and then regaining it
- frequently thinking about 'cutting down' on food or missing meals
- fearing starvation or deprivation
- missing a proper breakfast—a proper breakfast consists of at least a bowl of cereal that is low in fat and has no added sugar (do not count muffins, liquid replacements or food concentrates)
- feeling fat or ugly, or indeed having any negative feelings about your body
- being exposed to undue stress, worry or fear
- not sleeping properly (i.e. not getting eight hours of uninterrupted sleep per night, from which you wake feeling energised and refreshed)
- drinking insufficient water (at least 1 L and preferably 2 L per day)
- not making sure you have healthy snacks between meals
- not doing physical exercise every day
- allowing your muscles to waste away.

PART 1 UNDERSTANDING WHY YOU ARE OVERWEIGHT

Where do you start?

I know it probably looks rather daunting right now, but I'm not about to hold out on you. You need to know how to recognise a problem when you see it!

But guess what? You don't have to get all extreme about it. The fittest, healthiest people engage in lots of these unhealthy behaviours and they're still fit, slim and healthy.

How do they do it? The answer is moderation. Some of these problems may be quite big for you (one patient I treated was eating a minimum of one family-sized block of chocolate every day—and that was when they had it under control!). They're obviously the problems with the biggest impact and are the ones you need to concentrate on.

Notice that some of these problems could come under the heading 'habits' (like eating in front of the television), while others come under the heading 'emotional' (like eating because you feel sad). Different techniques work to eliminate different kinds of problems, as you'll see in Part 2.

So go easy on yourself, take it slowly and practise moderation. This is not a race to perfection, but a change in direction. You are moving towards health and wellbeing, and the changes you are making are not just the latest fad—because you are making real, deep changes at the level of your subconscious, they are changes for life.

Part 2
Techniques for effortless change

Chapter 5
The chocoholic workshop: food triggers to eating

Like Pavlov's dogs, we have all learned unconscious responses to the smell or sight of certain foods. Many of us are literally out of control because the food controls us instead of us controlling the food. Keep very much in mind as you work through this book that it is necessary that you eat and drink what you want. Deliberate dieting is not only counterproductive, but it also gives a false benchmark. Therefore, it is unnecessary to deprive yourself in order to normalise your weight (deprivation causes cravings). However, it is absolutely necessary that you recognise and admit to those things that have been in the way of reaching and living your goal, and are willing to apply treatment techniques to those things.

This chapter will help you to:
- ✓ Understand your food 'triggers'.
- ✓ Learn to use the NLP 'anchoring' technique to turn off the food triggers instantly and permanently.
- ✓ Learn to use the same NLP technique to make good food far more exciting.

PART 2 TECHNIQUES FOR EFFORTLESS CHANGE

Neuro-linguistic programming

Originally developed by American academics Richard Bandler and John Grinder, and now a vast field encompassing language and subjective experience, NLP can be thought of as the study of excellence in human performance.

NLP has been described in many different ways and this presents some controversy, depending on whether we call it a science, a field, a body of knowledge, a philosophy, a collection of observations or techniques, or an epistemology. If you have a working definition of NLP, you can rest assured that at least some of the world's most renowned NLP experts will probably disagree with you, as well as with each other.

For most of us who have definite, practical requirements from our study and practice of NLP, none of this may matter.

The term 'neuro-linguistic programming' was first coined by Bandler and Grinder as they continued the work of transformational grammarians in the late 1970s. NLP also grew out of 'modelling', the process of examining and interpreting the behaviour of 'excellence' so that excellence could be explained, taught and replicated. This is one aspect of NLP that has grown very little since the early days, apart from Bandler's development of Design Human Engineering™ and the work of a few creative pioneers, such as Rex Sikes, a master trainer based in the United States.

Initially, the models used were that of excellence in therapy, and we owe much of the content and philosophy of NLP to revered therapists such as Milton Erickson (Ericksonian hypnosis), Virginia Satir (family therapy), Fritz Perls (gestalt therapy) and Frank Farrelly (provocative therapy). These therapists were mostly unable to explain their own brilliance, since much that they did was below consciousness (perhaps in the nature of 'intuition'). However, when their performance was analysed by Bandler and Grinder, what had formerly been unconscious and unnoticed became available for us all.

One thing is for sure: NLP is not a magic wand. The classic NLP texts are full of amazing and miraculous stories, the 'myths and legends' of NLP, many of which do not fully 'check out'. NLP is, however, exceedingly useful, and will empower your communication

CHAPTER 5 FOOD TRIGGERS TO EATING

and your life in ways you never dreamed possible. In a therapeutic context, NLP skills give enormous advantage. In selling and persuasion, likewise.

It is probably best if you decide for yourself on a working definition for NLP.

Do you recognise yourself among Sarah, Janie and Margaret?

Sarah had a problem with chocolate—she couldn't just stop at a few pieces, she literally had to eat it until it was gone. Janie had a problem with bread—she could easily devour a whole loaf, especially a fresh French loaf slathered with butter! Margaret didn't have a problem with a particular food, but when she was tired, stressed or bored, she would find herself eating without even thinking about it. These women, like so many people, were simply eating too much.

While Janie and Margaret were overweight from their habits, Sarah was slim because she made up for the chocolate by cutting down on other food (and nutrition). These women were damaging their health. They also had in common a lot of guilt and shame over their eating, often eating in secret—for example, after the family had gone to bed, when they were alone in front of the television, when they were driving the car or even hiding behind the pantry door.

None of this was their fault! The reason for their eating behaviour was their unconscious mind. This is why willpower had never stood a chance!

Using techniques from neuro-linguistics, these women made changes that didn't depend on willpower. The Lifeworks Group helped them to actually change their subconscious programming so that their feelings about food became very different.

Sarah, for instance, discovered that she could still enjoy chocolate, but now without guilt—she simply didn't think about it that much. Janie now enjoyed a slice or two of bread and absolutely didn't desire any more—one or two was enough! Margaret no longer felt hungry when she found herself tired or stressed. She found herself changing her life for the better instead of putting up with it and using food as a comfort!

PART 2 TECHNIQUES FOR EFFORTLESS CHANGE

SOMETIMES FOOD SERVES A VERY IMPORTANT PURPOSE

I mean a purpose quite apart from fuel for your body! Sometimes, overeating is a sort of psychological survival technique.

WHAT HAPPENS IN MY 'BEAT CRAVINGS, SHIFT FAT!' WORKSHOPS

In my 'Beat cravings, shift fat!' workshops, when I get to the part where I explain food addiction as part of the complexity that makes up a weight problem, I ask the group to nominate a particular problem food. Typically, most people will say 'chocolate' (that's why many people call the workshop 'The chocoholic workshop').

Then I ask everyone what chocolate does for them. How do they feel just before they realise they 'need' it? How does it make them feel? What purpose does it serve? We end up with a diagram on the whiteboard that looks something like Figure 5.1. Often the list is quite long, and the participants begin to get an idea of the nature of the problems that chocolate currently serves to mask. They understand that there are problems in their lives that chocolate actually helps them to cope with. Chocolate carries a real weight!

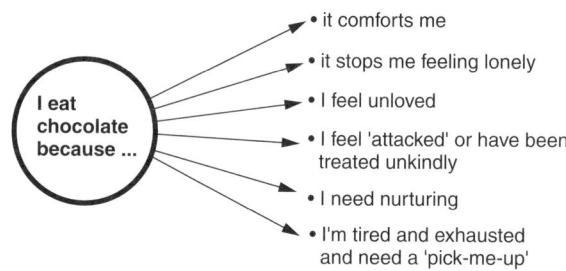

Figure 5.1 Chocolate may have non-food meanings that serve to comfort, nurture, reward or numb you

Then I ask, 'What would happen if I just took the chocolate away?' and I erase the word 'chocolate' from the whiteboard. Immediately, there are gasps around the room and many people are able to understand, not just logically, but from their gut, just how integral chocolate is for them.

CHAPTER 5 FOOD TRIGGERS TO EATING

Now the question is: 'Is it just a simple matter of removing my addiction?' Clearly, the answer is 'no'. If you simply remove the compulsion to eat chocolate, then you are left facing the problem with no 'anaesthetic'. Now nothing can numb you from the pain, unless of course you choose another anaesthetic.

When we see people hopping from one addictive substance to another, we say they have an 'addictive personality'. It is not their personality that is addictive, it is the lifestyle that screams out for something to numb the pain.

If you are working on your lifestyle, then you can indeed safely and comfortably use a variety of NLP techniques, or other rapid methods, to eliminate your food addiction. But if you try to deal with food addiction without considering these matters, it would be at best a waste of time, and at worst extremely distressful.

THIS SECTION MIGHT NOT APPLY TO YOU

If, from reading this chapter so far, you realise that it's not appropriate for you to treat food addictions or compulsions at this time, read through the rest of the chapter without actually doing the exercises and then obtain the expert assistance that you need to make positive changes for your health and wellbeing. You can still benefit from reading and doing the exercises in the remainder of the book.

However, if you know very well that chocolate or some other food serves an important function to numb your emotional pain, or to give you good feelings that are otherwise missing from your life, this is another matter altogether. You must look squarely at the facts beneath your addictive eating and be prepared to deal with them. You have at least three choices:

1. You can decide to deny or ignore your problems. If this is the way you want to go, then skip this whole chapter for now. You aren't ready and you aren't prepared. And this is not your fault—it's just the way things are for now.
2. If you feel that your problems are manageable with a bit of planning and commitment, then make a list of them and start working your way through them as you continue working with the book.
3. If you realise that your problems are big, or complex, then the best thing you can do is to get expert assistance from a licensed counsellor,

psychologist or psychiatrist. Brain surgeons do not generally operate on their own brain. You'd be expecting way too much of yourself to expect that you could deal with such big or complex issues while suffering in the midst of them. If you get the right help, you'll move through them a lot faster and a lot more comfortably than if you stay isolated. For some people, it may even be a good idea to put this whole book aside and deal with the more pressing issues first.

Let me give you an example of the last 'choice'. I had a client, Julie, who had come along to one of my workshops but had not used the techniques at all. She was disappointed enough by her 'self-sabotage' that she booked in for a therapy session in order to get to the bottom of it.

As we chatted it became obvious that Julie had far more than her weight to deal with. She literally didn't have a moment to herself throughout the day. She had three small children of school age, worked full-time and did all the housework including all cooking and cleaning. Her husband worked similar hours but did nothing around the house, even with the children. He was very demanding of her time and attention, and simultaneously verbally cruel and abusive. When she wasn't obedient, he would hit her. She learned to be very obedient. It didn't pay to even look unhappy with her lot.

So now, on top of all of this, Julie expected herself to commit to and use a program that would eliminate her food cravings. But even if she did have the time, taking away her food addictions would merely leave her without comfort in an incredibly harsh environment. So Julie's first priority had to be to sort out her home life. This was far too big, and possibly too dangerous, to handle alone, and Julie wisely elected to engage counselling support.

I really do urge you, if you have a similarly difficult situation to Julie, please nurture yourself by perhaps reading and enjoying this book, but more importantly by getting the assistance you deserve to create a better life for you and your family.

TRIGGERS TO EATING

On the understanding that any underlying life issues or problems are being dealt with appropriately, you are now ready to look at the triggering mechanisms that in the past have automatically flung you into eating behaviour that was out of your control.

CHAPTER 5 FOOD TRIGGERS TO EATING

A trigger is any sensory stimulus that sets off an automatic response and can be from any sensory representational system: visual, auditory, kinaesthetic, olfactory or gustatory. In NLP, we call these triggers 'anchors'. We each already have a lot of these anchors, in all sensory systems:

System	Examples
Visual (sight)	Your partner gives you 'that look' and you immediately respond with emotion. Someone holds out their hand and you automatically reach out to shake it.
Auditory (sound)	You hear an old song from your teenage years and are immediately transported back to that time. The phone rings and you jump to answer it.
Kinaesthetic (emotion/ body)	The feeling of mud between your toes automatically gives rise to feelings of delight or revulsion. A limp handshake automatically makes your stomach 'churn'.
Olfactory (smell)	You get a certain feeling when you smell fresh-baked bread. A perfume reminds you straight away of someone.
Gustatory (taste)	Someone bakes a pie for you 'just like Mum used to make' and as you take a bite you get an automatic feeling that goes with it. You bite into an orange and your lips swell up because when you were a child you bit an orange with a wasp on it and got bitten in turn!

You collect these anchors your whole life, although probably the most powerful were collected when you were very young. Here is an example of a kinaesthetic anchor that still works for you, even though it was created when you were probably under the age of seven. Try it out!

EXERCISE

While sitting, have a friend pat you on the head, chuck you under the chin or squeeze your cheek. Now, no-one has done that to you for probably decades, but the feelings are still there, aren't they?

So, you have anchors or triggers that 'fire' when you see, hear, taste, smell or touch certain things, sometimes even when that is only in your imagination! They got there 'by accident' as you went about your life, learning and experiencing. They got there because your mind 'associated' a certain event with a certain emotional state.

Now that you understand that, you can make use of the same mechanism to quite deliberately install your own anchors and use them to your advantage. The process of installing and using anchors is called 'anchoring'. The uses of anchoring are limited only by your imagination.

In this book I'm going to teach you how to use kinaesthetic anchors in a very special way. The process is called 'collapse anchors' and although it has a multitude of uses, I'll be showing you how to use 'collapse anchors' to turn off your cravings for unhealthy food choices and to turn on some cravings for healthy food and exercise choices. This is how you get your unconscious mind to do the work for you!

THE COLLAPSE ANCHORS TECHNIQUE

In this technique I'll teach you to install two kinaesthetic anchors, one on the left knee and one on the right. If you do this properly, when you touch one knee you'll get a particular feeling, and when you touch the other knee you'll get a very different feeling.

For instance, you might install an anchor that is associated with chocolate (or another craving) on one knee and an anchor that is associated with the thought of drinking blended raw snails on the other knee. As you might imagine, if you've been successful, as you fire the anchor on each knee, you'll get a very different feeling.

Once these two anchors are successfully installed on your knees, we'll then 'collapse' them by firing them together in the right sequence. If you complete this stage successfully, you'll be unable to get excited about what was previously a craving.

Don't worry, you'll still be able to eat and enjoy that food, it's just that now it will be by choice, not because you feel compelled! All that awful 'neediness' around the particular food will be gone and you'll feel quite detached and free about it.

CHAPTER 5 FOOD TRIGGERS TO EATING

THE IMPORTANCE OF PRECISION

There are three things to remember in setting anchors: precision, precision and precision!

You need to set the anchor in the same physical location on your body, with the same intensity, with the same duration, at just the moment you are coming towards the 'peak' of the state you wish to anchor. Make sure you touch exactly the same spot (you could use a chalk mark, a spot on a seam or even a freckle) with the same intensity (a stronger touch does not mean it sets 'harder'!) and for exactly the same time duration.

The reason we set anchors as we are coming into the peak of a state, rather than at the peak, is that internal states tend to drop away very quickly once the peak of the state is actually reached. Do you really want to anchor 'dropping away'? Then make sure that you set your anchor as you are coming into the peak of the state.

SETTING UP

You are going to set two kinaesthetic anchors—one that triggers feelings that match your feelings about a certain food, and one that triggers feelings that match your feelings about something that disgusts you. Then you are going to collapse these two anchors into each other with the process called, naturally, 'collapse anchors'.

The result of this, if done correctly, is that when you think about the food, or are presented with it, you'll now feel something ranging between neutral and disgust. Don't be concerned if you feel real disgust for the food you used to go ape over—that feeling will fade back within a few days and become quite neutral. You will still enjoy that food now and again, guilt free, and it will no longer control you.

To set the anchor, you need to get into a relaxed position with your fingertips poised to touch your kneecap as you approach the peak of the feeling you want to anchor. (There is nothing magical about kneecaps—you could use ear lobes or just touch fingertips together and it would work just as well.)

Sit relaxed with your arms resting along the tops of your legs, the heels of your hands resting just above your knees and your fingertips poised to anchor the two feelings (see Figure 5.2). Using this position means that each time you touch against your kneecap it will be in exactly the same place, for exactly the same duration, with exactly the same intensity. You may like to close your eyes to aid your concentration. However, some people concentrate better with their eyes open.

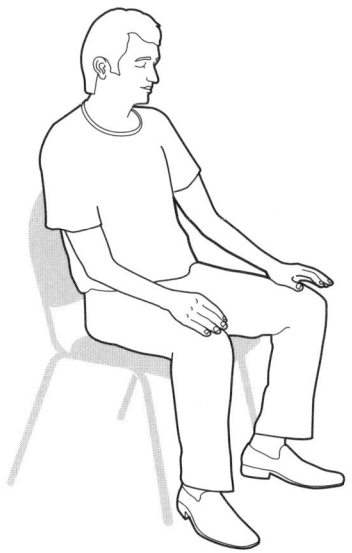

Figure 5.2 The 'ready' position for setting up kinaesthetic anchors, using the kneecaps

In the following exercise you'll choose a particular food that you agree you eat too much of or that you may even obsess over. You will notice the feelings you get when you vividly imagine eating this food, and you will set an anchor for those feelings on your left knee. You'll also choose a substance that is particularly revolting to you and you'll notice the feelings you get when you vividly imagine being close to or even tasting this substance. You'll set an anchor for these feelings on your right knee. Finally, you'll collapse these anchors together, permanently gaining freedom from the food that once was a problem for you.

EXERCISE: TREATING A CHOCOLATE ADDICTION

Note: you'll need undisturbed time and perhaps even a friend to help pace you through the steps.

1. Imagine yourself eating a specific type of chocolate—for example, Cadbury's Dairy Milk, a Mars Bar or Classic Tim

CHAPTER 5 FOOD TRIGGERS TO EATING

Tams. It must be a specific type of chocolate to work properly. By the time you've treated three to five specific types of chocolate in the same way, the effect will generalise across all types of chocolate. However, if you treat just 'chocolate' generally, it is unlikely to be as effective.

As you feel yourself really getting into all the sensory stuff around eating chocolate (the smell, the first bite, the smoothness, the meltingness, etc.) bring your fingertips to your left knee for two seconds. Then raise your fingertips from your knee and quickly 'break state' by opening your eyes and concentrating on something neutral (e.g. look out of the window at something, count backwards from 20 in three's or think of a flower).

Repeat this exact process twice more.

2. From a neutral state, bring your fingertips to your left knee in the same way as before, without trying to think about the chocolate. If you have been successful, you will immediately feel the same effects as though you were thinking about the chocolate and this will probably be quite definite physical feelings—for example, a feeling in your stomach or chest area, salivation or a 'smiley' feeling perhaps. If you have been successful, you can move on to step 3. If not, you must repeat steps 1 and 2.

3. Imagine something so disgusting to you that there is no way you would put it anywhere near your mouth. Some people use food that they hate, and almost every nurse I've taught this technique to has used the thought of sputum. Imagine this thing very vividly—the more intense the better—and even imagine what it might taste like!

As you feel the disgust, bring your other fingertips to your right knee for two seconds. Then raise your fingertips and quickly break state exactly as before.

Warning! Do not use things you are afraid of, or things that are linked to real-life sadness or distress. Do I need to spell out why? You absolutely do not want to trigger genuine fear states because of the risk of distress, and in any case NLP is not about 'walking over broken glass' in order to get the changes you desire. It is about investigating and developing efficient, elegant ways to achieve change automatically and naturally.

Repeat this exact process twice more.
4. From a neutral state, bring your fingertips to your right knee in the same way as before, without trying to think of the 'disgusting' thing. If you have been successful, you will immediately get that same physical sense of revulsion and can move on to step 5. If not, you must repeat steps 3 and 4.
5. From a neutral state, fire the 'chocolate' anchor by bringing your fingertips to your left knee in the same way as before, only this time say to yourself 'And put that over the top of it'. As you say the word 'that', bring your other fingertips to your right knee.

You may feel a sense of confusion or spaciness, or you may even get a physical 'butterflies' type feeling around the midline of your body. This is a sign that the anchors are certainly collapsing and at this point say to yourself 'That's right'. Then raise your fingers from the chocolate anchor and, after two seconds, raise your fingers from the 'disgust' anchor and quickly break state exactly as before.

Repeat this exact process twice more.
6. With the 'disgust' anchor activated (touched), think of your specific chocolate and try to get interested in it. This should fail.
7. With the 'chocolate' anchor activated (touched), think of your specific chocolate and try to get interested in it. This should also fail.

This process should be used to treat every non-healthy food you can think of, as well as healthy foods that you eat too much of. How much is too much? Check Chapter 17 to find out!

Adding oomph to healthy food:
Using the pleasure principle

What is it that makes some things utterly irresistible? So utterly irresistible that if someone asks us whether or not we want it, we don't even hesitate to answer, we just automatically reach out and take it!

CHAPTER 5 FOOD TRIGGERS TO EATING

Perhaps there are no words to describe that intense feeling of utter desire and pleasure that surrounds the irresistible thing. Usually the feeling is so visceral that it is beyond words. What do you have, or have you had, in your life that evokes those feelings for you?

Imagine what it would be like to take those wantonly wonderful feelings and copy them across to things or activities that you'd like to feel really, really good about but don't just yet. Imagine what it would be like to:

- feel warm and wonderful about low-fat cereal
- feel excited about fruit
- feel orgasmic about salads
- feel sheer, unmitigated pleasure while shopping for and preparing healthy food.

Can you guess how you can use the collapse anchors technique to achieve all this easily and automatically? In the following exercise, you'll anchor the 'good' food feeling (which is not yet a 'great' feeling for you) on your left knee and then anchor the 'extreme pleasure' feeling on your right knee. When you collapse these two sets of feelings together, the result is a far more positive attitude towards healthy food. You'll notice that you don't have to talk yourself into this improved attitude because the feeling is very genuine!

EXERCISE

So now, anchor the thought of the specific cereal, fruit or salad, or the thought of shopping for or preparing these things, on your left knee, and the thought of the thing you feel ecstatic about on your right knee, using exactly the same technique as before:

1. As you feel yourself really getting into all the sensory stuff around eating the healthy food, bring your fingertips to your left knee for two seconds. Then raise your fingertips from your knee and quickly break state by opening your eyes and concentrating on something neutral.
    Repeat this exact process twice more.
2. From a neutral state, bring your fingertips to your left knee in the same way as before, without trying to think about

that food. If you have been successful, you will immediately feel the same effects as though you were thinking about the food and this will mean definite physical feelings. If you have been successful, you can move on to step 3. If not, you must repeat steps 1 and 2.

3. Imagine something so ecstatically wonderful that even now, just thinking about it, you feel warm and excited. Imagine this thing very vividly—the more intense the better.

   As you feel yourself coming towards the peak of this feeling, bring your other fingertips to your right knee for two seconds. Then raise your fingertips and quickly break state exactly as before.

   Repeat this exact process twice more.

4. From a neutral state, bring your fingertips to your right knee in the same way as before, without trying to think of the 'wonderful' thing. If you have been successful, you will immediately get that same physical sense of warmth and excitement and can move on to step 5. If not, you must repeat steps 3 and 4.

5. From a neutral state, fire the 'healthy food' anchor by bringing your fingertips to your left knee in the same way as before, only this time say to yourself 'And put that over the top of it'. As you say the word 'that', bring your other fingertips to your right knee.

   With both sets of fingertips in the anchor position, say to yourself 'That's right'. Then raise your fingers from the 'healthy food' anchor and, after two seconds, raise your fingers from the 'wonderful' anchor and quickly break state exactly as before.

   Repeat this exact process twice more.

6. With the 'wonderful' anchor activated (touched), think of your specific healthy food and check how you feel about it. It should feel rather nice! Just to check, break state for a moment and then think of the specific healthy food without firing the anchor. It should still feel rather nice.

So you first learned how to use collapse anchors as an 'aversion' technique. Now you've learned how to use it as an 'attraction' technique. Are you getting the idea of how versatile this incredible technique actually is?

You now know that you already have kinaesthetic anchors, and you've learned how to install and manipulate your own. How can you make use of an auditory anchor you already have?

An auditory anchor you already have: the yummy noise factor

Many people are aware that we make mental pictures, sounds, tastes, smells and feelings inside our own heads as we go about our lives day to day. Few people are aware that we can manipulate these internal representations in order to dramatically alter our perception of the world and indeed our experience of reality itself.

Exercise

Next time you're eating a food that you'd like to enjoy more, experiment with making 'yummy noises' as you eat: 'Mmmm!' What difference does that make?

Next time you think of salad, what happens when you turn up the colours, big and bright in your head, and use a moving picture, like a video, instead of just a still picture?

When you're shopping, how much more enjoyable could it be with a gorgeously seductive voice whispering in your ear 'Look at those mouth-watering grapes!' If you've never had the fruit and vegetable section talk to you, you don't know what you've been missing!

How much more delight and pleasure can you bring to your daily life? How much delight can you stand?

Chapter 6
Excuses, excuses!
Attitude to exercise

For many people, their exercise needs have been ignored for years. The pressures of work, family responsibilities, stress and exhaustion have all taken their toll and prevented them from taking the time they need to care for their bodies. Now is the time to get your life back and do nice things for your body so that your body does nice things for you.

This chapter will help you to:

✓ Understand all the fuss about exercise.

✓ Find great ways to start moving, even if you're a beginner.

✓ Love the feeling of moving your body.

CHAPTER 6 ATTITUDE TO EXERCISE

MEET THE BLOB

Figure 6.1 shows one of my pet props, the famous blob, just 2.3 kg of it. And in case you think it looks unrealistic, think again! This is what human fat looks like. Notice it has hardly any blood supply, just a few scant capillaries on the outside. Muscles, on the other hand, require a rich blood supply to function, burning up fat and increasing our metabolic rate.

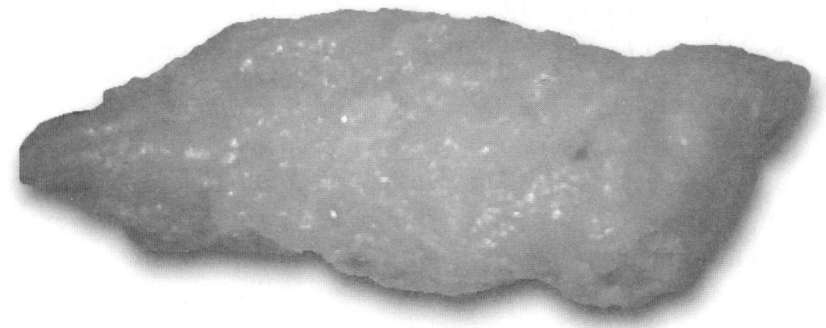

Figure 6.1 2.3 kg of human fat looks just like this!

The excess fat that you have is exactly like this. One woman who attended my clinic said that a group she was with had been horrified when an overweight friend was bitten by a dog, lacerating her arm, and bright yellow globs of fat popped out from the laceration.

It certainly is scary to think that some of us carry a pillow-sized layer (or thicker) of this bright yellow stuff, completely encasing our bodies, stretching our poor skin out of all proportion! Not to mention the diabetes, heart disease, joint deterioration and arthritis, gall bladder disease, varicose veins, gout, respiratory problems and several types of cancer that are all directly attributable to being overweight.

Our hospitals are literally clogged with patients who are suffering from the many complications of obesity, and no government can afford to continue propping up a healthcare system that is merely reacting to self-abuse. Doctors estimate that over 60 per cent of the illnesses and diseases they treat daily in their surgeries are directly caused by inactivity! In Australia, roughly 20 per cent of all deaths in hospitals are directly attributable to people being overweight.

We need to do something about our bodies now, not only for ourselves and our own health, but for our children's health and for the economic salvation of the entire healthcare system!

You've begun to deal with food addictions and compulsions, now you're ready to deal with every single thing that is in the way of your absolutely loving the feeling of your body in movement!

Focus on physical movement

If you do not undertake physical exercise regularly and sufficiently to keep your body in good health, you will suffer a range of serious health effects:

- Your lymphatic system will not work properly, leading to a build-up of poisonous 'stuff' that really shouldn't be in your body. The lymphatic system is vital for removing waste, toxins and excess fluid from your body. Unlike the pulmonary system, the lymphatic system has no 'pump'—it is activated purely by muscle movement!
- Your muscles will waste away, decreasing your metabolic rate.
- You will lose fitness, making everyday 'getting around' so much more difficult and tiring.
- You won't be able to do basic things like gardening, or playing with children, because of your lack of fitness and deterioration of strength.
- You won't get enough oxygen moving through your body and you will begin to experience confusion, even short-term memory loss.
- Your circulation will become impaired.
- Your blood pressure will increase.
- Your immune system and other systems will suffer.
- Your sleep will suffer.
- You will feel generally tired, low in energy and unwell. You might have that 'hit by a truck' feeling when you wake up in the morning.
- You might become quite depressed.
- Healthy people will find you boring and tedious to be with because you are so sluggish.

Even if you lose weight without exercise, just by altering your food tastes, you will not have good health. Your body was designed to move and your muscles were designed to be challenged. If you don't do enough of that, you are actually engaging in self-abuse!

CHAPTER 6 ATTITUDE TO EXERCISE

So many mental and physical disorders are directly caused by lack of activity, and expecting to be healthy without exercise is just as senseless as expecting to remain well while drinking a bucket of petrol (gasoline, for our American readers) every day! Death rates from inactivity are greater than those from smoking and unsafe sex combined!

You don't have to force yourself to do boring physical activity, or activity that feels like 'punishment'. This is definitely counterproductive to the whole program. If you embark on an exercise program by using willpower, as you have no doubt done before, you know it won't last.

Australian health department studies show that while people who diet regain the weight within three years, people who lose weight through exercise alone regain it in just 12 months! So, while you need to exercise in order to lose weight and be healthy, you must also attend to the emotional reasons that prevent you from loving the feeling of moving your body, so that 'getting out to play' at every opportunity becomes a lifelong habit.

WHAT TYPE OF EXERCISE?

Let's start by considering what exercise you will do. There is little to be gained from attempting to commit to an activity that you consider to be boring. When you are seeking physical activity to increase your sense of wellbeing, think back to what you used to really enjoy earlier in life. Identify an exercise or sport that you can do purely for the pleasure of it, at least three times each week.

Special mention needs to be made about swimming, which is an excellent cardiovascular/aerobic activity. While swimming can indeed be regarded as one of the best exercises you can do, it's not generally considered to be a weight-loss activity. Sports physiotherapists say this is for two reasons: swimming both increases appetite and decreases metabolism as a reaction to the coolness of the water. If you choose swimming as your sport, make sure you combine it with land exercise.

Also be aware that slow walking is not a weight-reduction activity—nor is housework, light gardening and most forms of physical work. A relaxed game of tennis doubles is not a weight-reduction activity. These are all tremendously great starter activities for people with extremely low levels of fitness, but you'll soon need to ramp it up!

In addition to aerobic activity, you need to choose a type of resistance training that you also find interesting. This could be fitball, resistance

PART 2 TECHNIQUES FOR EFFORTLESS CHANGE

bands, free weights, gym equipment, or a combination of these. You will need to get proper advice about the correct way to use equipment because poor technique can be totally ineffective at best, and at worst even quite dangerous.

The following activities/sports are wonderful weight-reduction and fitness activities:

- ❏ walking at least 6 to 8 km/h (you should be able to hold a conversation, taking a breath every few words; use a talking pedometer if you want an easy measuring method—these can be purchased from Walk With Attitude! at *www.walkingwithattitude.com*, where you'll also find an incredible amount of resources for physical fitness)
- ❏ weight-resistance training (e.g. weights, resistance bands)
- ❏ fitball (for stabilisation, strength, balance)
- ❏ tennis (singles)
- ❏ touch football (fairly constant running—no long breaks)
- ❏ hockey (fairly constant running—no long breaks)
- ❏ squash (constant play for at least two 15-minute sessions)
- ❏ aerobics
- ❏ treadmill
- ❏ circuit training
- ❏ rollerblading (the Morley rollerbladers are aged 70 and above!)
- ❏ cycling (constant, not coasting downhill!)
- ❏ stair or step climbing
- ❏ pump classes
- ❏ beach walking
- ❏ kickboxing
- ❏ Yogacise or Ashtunga Yoga
- ❏ Pilates.

It's important to include some type of muscle resistance activity because increased muscle mass automatically increases your metabolism, helping to burn excess fat.

USING ANCHORING TO ENHANCE YOUR EXERCISE PLEASURE

This is the NLP collapse anchors technique that you learned to use as an 'attraction' therapy in Chapter 5.

EXERCISE

1. Just as you did in Chapter 5, set an anchor on your left knee representing the exercise you want to feel excited about. To do this, you need to vividly imagine yourself engaged in the activity. For example, if the activity is brisk walking, mentally engage all your senses to imagine being out brisk walking. Feel your arms and legs pumping and the oxygen coursing through your body. Feel the breeze on your face and in your hair and cooling the heat that is building up as you work out. You might, if you visualise well, imagine what you would see on your walk. Perhaps you'd imagine certain sounds and smells as well. As you feel yourself coming into the peak of the experience, quickly anchor this on your left knee and then break state as before.
   Repeat this exact process twice more.
2. Now test that the anchor is working. You won't necessarily think 'walking' when you fire the anchor, but you should get some of the same physical sensations as you did when imagining it.
3. Now it's time to anchor a feeling that you could describe as 'ecstatic' on the right knee. Choose something that you find intensely exciting—perhaps the thought of winning the lottery or winning a prize, or the best sex you've ever had!
   Repeat this exact process twice more.
4. Again, test that the anchor is working.
5. Now collapse anchors just as you did in Chapter 5. First fire the 'exercise' anchor and then two seconds later fire the 'ecstatic' anchor, saying to yourself as you do so 'And put that over the top of it'. Take off the 'exercise' anchor first, followed two seconds later by the 'ecstatic' anchor and quickly break state.
   Repeat this exact process twice more.

Many people have found it helpful to collapse anchors with something far from ecstatic! It may seem strange to you, but the state or feeling of brushing your teeth is often very effective to collapse over the top of an 'exercise' state. This is because for many people brushing their teeth:

PART 2 TECHNIQUES FOR EFFORTLESS CHANGE

- is absolutely routine
- is something they wouldn't think of starting the day without it
- is something they might do more than once a day if they feel like it
- feels nice and refreshing while they're doing it
- gives them an 'aaahhhhh' feeling immediately afterwards.

Which is all good stuff to associate with exercise, don't you think? What other feelings might combine well with exercise?

LOVE THE FEELING OF BEING AWARE OF YOUR BODY!

You've used anchoring to add oomph to foods and food activity. Now it's time to use this principle to enjoy the feeling of being in your own body, and in particular to enjoy the feeling of strong muscles moving under your skin, helping to burn that excess fat and adding to your feeling of energy and wellbeing.

Your job now is to fire your 'ecstatic' anchor whenever you become aware of muscle strength and whenever you think of or do physical exercise.

Imagine how it will be to feel those wantonly wonderful feelings whenever you:

- lift something and feel your arm and leg muscles tensing
- walk slowly or quickly
- go up or down stairs
- stretch
- stand up from a chair
- exert yourself to the point of perspiration.

Isn't this so much better than before, when you were almost unconscious of your poor body and just sort of dragged it around from day to day? Now, when you sense the feeling of really 'being in your body', you want to ensure that it's accompanied by a feeling of energy and exhilaration!

It's also time to get selfish about taking time to maintain, nurture and care for your body. Your body has to last you the rest of your life and you want to make sure it can go the distance and maintain its health and vitality.

There are two ways you can do this.

CHAPTER 6 ATTITUDE TO EXERCISE

1. Activities that create fitness, strength and vitality
   - ☐ Schedule in a physical activity daily—30–60 minutes of brisk walking is highly recommended.
   - ☐ Schedule in an exercise or sport three times per week—tennis, aerobics, yoga, touch football, kickboxing and tai chi are all excellent.
   - ☐ Schedule in resistance activities such as fitball, sculpting bands or weights.

2. Activities that provide a delicious sense of nurture and enhance wellbeing

   Schedule in a 'spoiling' session at least once a week:
   - ☐ a bubble bath/spa
   - ☐ a manicure/pedicure
   - ☐ a massage
   - ☐ a visit to the hairdresser
   - ☐ a whole hour reading outside under a tree
   - ☐ a stroll along a beach.

   There are an infinite number of ways you can treat yourself. Sex is a great way to get exercise and nurture all in one! Did you know, for instance, that a very active lovemaking session can use up the same amount of kilojoules as running up and down 368 steps!

SPECIAL NOTE

If you don't think you have time to exercise, there's something seriously wrong with your life. That's like saying 'I don't have time to eat' or 'I don't have time to breathe'. Certainly, there are times in your life, times of crisis, when you have to put all else aside and make some fairly significant sacrifices. But when this situation continues indefinitely, it is absolutely unacceptable and you need to do whatever it takes to ensure your health and wellbeing!

Likewise, some people may think that they have a health reason for avoiding exercise. They may have a poor heart or a disability that greatly restricts movement. But they can still do something, albeit only after following expert advice to ensure that they can exercise safely and within their capabilities. Even someone who is completely immobile can do the breathing exercises from Qi Gong, for instance.

Chapter 7
Eating when you're not hungry: emotional triggers to eating

Even after you've eliminated compulsions and addictions about certain foods, you may still find that you engage in 'non-hungry' eating. This also needs attention if you are to gain free will over what you eat and when you eat.

This chapter will help you to:

✓ Understand the role of your emotions in eating behaviour.

✓ Use the amazing resource triangle, an NLP technique that can stop any negative emotion in its tracks!

CHAPTER 7 EMOTIONAL TRIGGERS TO EATING

The emotions that lead you to eat

Most of us have particular states of mind (emotional or psychological) that trigger us to eat. You might be able to control them for a short time, but inevitably they will win out, driving you to demolish a whole packet of biscuits instead of stopping at just one, or driving you to eat guiltily behind the pantry door as you bust out of your diet and don't want anyone to know.

It's important to remember that these emotions are not 'you'—they're just programmed responses that you've built up over the years in order to deal with life. You could say that these sorts of emotions are just 'bad programming'.

But don't be too hard on these emotions. They didn't get programmed into your brain in order to give you a hard time! They got programmed in because your brain treated them as a useful response to a particular event. For instance, if, when you were a child, your mother gave you chocolate or some other sweet thing to soothe you, it is highly likely that you will now regard that food as a 'comfort' food and automatically reach for it when you feel lonely or sad. It's not that you *decided* that chocolate equals comfort—your brain automatically interpreted it that way on your behalf! It's not the past *event* that is the problem, it is your *perception* of it and the automatic programming that was set in place at the time.

People engage in non-hungry eating for many reasons:

- tiredness
- boredom
- sadness/depression
- anger
- fear
- stress
- loneliness
- reward
- comfort/solace
- celebration.

And these feelings may be triggered by situations such as:

- driving home
- watching television
- having an argument
- walking through the front door
- seeing the refrigerator/pantry
- watching others eat.

All these triggers, emotional and situational, are perfect fodder for the resource triangle!

PART 2 TECHNIQUES FOR EFFORTLESS CHANGE

Case Studies

Case 1: Rebecca couldn't stop buying chocolate on her way home from work

Rebecca reported always having to buy a chocolate bar from the corner deli on her way home from work. This was an automatic behaviour pattern and was very entrenched. Rebecca had tried to stop herself but the feelings she got about 'missing out' or 'being deprived' were so strong that she literally couldn't help herself. In fact, the more she tried to deprive herself, the greater was her craving!

I asked Rebecca to relax and describe the process of finishing work and driving home, stopping at several points to check whether the 'chocolate' feeling was there. For instance, when I asked 'And as you get up to leave your desk, is the chocolate feeling there?' and 'And when you get into your car in the car park, is the chocolate feeling there?', she answered quite confidently 'No, it isn't'. In fact, we discovered that Rebecca would get the 'chocolate' feeling when she reached a certain point on her journey home.

This was great news, because we had identified the key point, the turning point, in the unconscious program that controlled Rebecca's behaviour. We could take that key point and alter the meaning of it so that it no longer led to chocolate. We used the resource triangle, which you'll learn about shortly, and Rebecca suddenly started 'forgetting' to stop for chocolate on the way home.

Case 2: Mandy got the munchies after dinner each night

Mandy had a problem with snacking after dinner. She was eating well throughout the day and made sure she ate the right food often enough. This meant that her evening snacking was most unlikely to be a result of low blood sugar or some other chemical reason. The reason looked like being an emotional one.

CHAPTER 7 EMOTIONAL TRIGGERS TO EATING

Mandy's routine was that she would bath and feed the children, then put them to bed and clear away the dinner things and toys. She would then 'collapse' onto the sofa in front of the television, where she would get a 'collapsed/bored' feeling, quickly followed by the urge to get something to eat while she watched television. For Mandy, that 'collapsed/bored' feeling was the key point, the turning point, which led to the poor eating behaviour.

We treated the 'collapsed/bored' feeling using the resource triangle and Mandy suddenly 'changed her mind' about the way she structured her evenings. Food no longer figured and she developed a variety of ways to relax and enjoy the peace and quiet. Mandy had broken the association between 'collapsed/bored' and food.

THE RESOURCE TRIANGLE

The technique I often use for this type of situation is the NLP technique called the resource triangle. This brilliant technique is possibly the most powerful and useful technique ever devised in the whole history of NLP!

The resource triangle is an exercise that starts off with you thinking very, very briefly about something that bothers you or that tends to launch you into unhelpful behaviour such as comfort eating or self-neglect. That something might be:

- a negative thought about yourself (e.g. 'I'm a failure')
- the sound of someone criticising you (e.g. a friend saying 'You never stick at anything')
- the thought of the clock reading 5.00 pm (because every day at that time you get an urge to eat rubbish)
- the stressed feeling you get right after dinner when you're tired and you realise that you still have so much to do (because that's when you eat chocolate, both for comfort and as an energy hit to get you through till bedtime).

The resource triangle takes that thought or feeling and over the space of around 15 minutes totally eliminates its emotional impact. As a result, the thought fades away or you find you simply cannot get the feeling back, even if you try!

When you are ready to use the resource triangle, you'll need to go through the detailed instructions opposite. However, to follow is a brief description (from which, for brevity, I've omitted some very important things you must do and say) so that you get an overall feel for how the resource triangle works.

1. Think of the thing (thought, feeling) that you want to eliminate and immediately break that state by thinking of something neutral (perhaps by counting backwards).
2. Think of something that you can imagine quite vividly (like a beach scene, the feeling of being in a spa, your favourite holiday destination, etc). The feeling you get from imagining this is called the 'resource state'.
3. Now combine the resource state with the old, bothersome feeling, so that the two really mix together. For instance, if your original thought was 'I'm a failure', and in step 2 you were imagining standing on a balcony in Broome enjoying a sunset, you would now, from your balcony in Broome, think to yourself 'I'm a failure'.
4. Repeat these three steps over and over again, each time using a different resource state. You will know when you are through when the original thought or feeling seems silly or meaningless and you are unable to get it back, even if you try.

Many people are amazed that by simply combining different feelings with a bothersome feeling, in a precise way, even extreme feelings can be eliminated easily and comfortably.

You can use the resource triangle to treat any negative feelings whatsoever that you may have about almost anything. I've even used it to eliminate severe phobias and clinical depression!

For NLPers, you might notice that the resource triangle uses anchoring, Ericksonian language, state management and conversational timeline all in one elegant package. No wonder it's so effective!

This deceptively simple floor exercise requires some skill in state management, as well as enough discipline to avoid any analytical thought whatsoever *during* the exercise. (Although, of course, analysis or evaluation *afterwards* may be most enlightening!) The technique also includes two particularly clever NLP language patterns (which you can learn more about later if you choose to study NLP and gain some facility with the meta model and the Milton Model).

CHAPTER 7 EMOTIONAL TRIGGERS TO EATING

Exercise: If you're stuck, move!
The amazing resource triangle

Make sure you've identified the problem thought or state before you commence the exercise. When you do step 1, you'll need to be prepared to literally think the thought or imagine the negative feeling you want to eliminate. If it is a feeling, you will have to identify the 'trigger' that gives you the negative feeling. From reading about anchoring, you'll appreciate that this trigger may be something you see (the clock), something you hear (a friend criticising you), something you feel (tired at the end of the day), something you smell (onions frying) or something you taste (chocolate).

To use the resource triangle, arrange three pieces of paper (one marked with an 'S', one marked with a 'D' and one marked with an 'R') in a triangle on the floor, as shown in Figure 7.1. The 'S' stands for 'stuck' and represents the feeling that you wish to eliminate; the 'D' stands for 'detached' or 'dissociated' and represents a neutral feeling; and the 'R' stands for 'resource' and represents (in turn) five or six different intense states that will be mingled with the 'S' feeling.

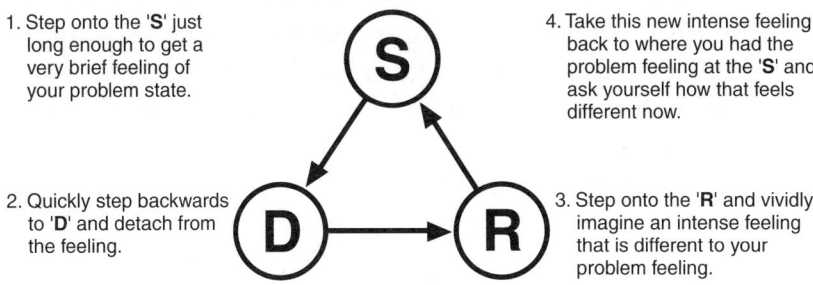

1. Step onto the '**S**' just long enough to get a very brief feeling of your problem state.

2. Quickly step backwards to '**D**' and detach from the feeling.

3. Step onto the '**R**' and vividly imagine an intense feeling that is different to your problem feeling.

4. Take this new intense feeling back to where you had the problem feeling at the '**S**' and ask yourself how that feels different now.

Figure 7.1 The resource triangle

On no account should you attempt to analyse the experience while stepping around the resource triangle. Do that later if you wish, but keep in mind that this is a process for the unconscious mind, not the conscious mind.

Work your way through the steps that follow.

PART 2 TECHNIQUES FOR EFFORTLESS CHANGE

1. Step onto the 'S', but be sure that you stand there only long enough to get the beginning 'trigger' of the feeling that you have been experiencing as a problem.
2. *Quickly* step backwards onto the 'D' and dissociate (detach from) the feeling you are freeing yourself from.
   To detach quickly, you could try a number of different techniques:
   - Imagine that you've left yourself standing on the 'S' and observe the back of yourself, watching yourself breathe.
   - Imagine that you are in a bubble or have a thick Perspex sheet between you and the 'S'.
   - Quickly count back from 20 in threes.
   - Gaze out of the window and 'make a shape' out of the first cloud you see.
3. While standing on the 'D', *decide* which resource state you wish to make use of *before* you step onto the 'R', then step onto the 'R'.
   The resource state does not have to be a positive state—it can be a very negative one. The important thing is that it is an *intense* state that you can access with relative ease, and also that it is very *different* from the target state you are wishing to eliminate. (That is, if you are intending to deal with a feeling of sadness, it could well be unhelpful to use 'anger' as a resource state. However, if you are intending to deal with a feeling of shyness, 'anger' could be useful.)
   Try these:
   - the experience of lying or walking on a beautiful beach
   - the experience of feeling intense awe
   - the experience of walking through putrid mud
   - the experience of being in a spa (make it fantastic!)
   - the experience of being acutely embarrassed
   - the experience of doing something exhilarating (paragliding?)
   - the experience of desperation (drowning? needing to get to a toilet? falling?)
   - any bizarre or disgusting experience (see the chicken leg fantasy below).

CHAPTER 7 EMOTIONAL TRIGGERS TO EATING

The chicken leg fantasy

Imagine that you are standing with a big, fat, warm, cooked chicken leg in each hand. Mmmmmm. And imagine that you take first one, and then the other, and gently insert them into each ear (have a yuuuuck tonality in your voice now and mimic the movements of inserting the chicken legs). And it's sort of greasy and yucky as you feel the warmth against your cheeks and smell that greasy cooked chicken smell and ... oh no, it's reeeaaalllly greasy and it's starting to drip, drip, drip down your shoulders and down your front (put a really disgusted look on your face as you gingerly lift your shirt outwards away from the 'grease') and it's sticking to your shirt and it's slowly congealing into a cold, sticky mass of chicken fat around the waistband of your trousers. Yuck!

See, it doesn't have to be a positive state to work really well.

4. Really intensify whatever resource state you are using. As you reach the *height* of that state, tell yourself 'Wrap this feeling all around me and **take that back** [and move back to the 'S'] **to where I had that problem feeling**', mix the old feeling and the new feeling together and say to yourself, 'How does that **feel differently now**?'. Take special note of the importance of the verbal instructions to your unconscious mind, particularly the parts in bold print. These are important language patterns and there is much more going on here than you might at first think!
5. Repeat this process several times, each time applying a different resource state. The more you vary the resource state, the faster and more powerful the effect.

SO WHAT DO YOU THINK OF FOR THE 'S'?

Deciding what to think of for the 'S' is the most important question you could possibly ask. Look at the following sequences of behaviour and note where the trigger points occur. It is the trigger point that needs to be identified.

PART 2 TECHNIQUES FOR EFFORTLESS CHANGE

- *Rebecca:* Tidy desk at end of day > leave office and walk to car park > get in car and start drive home > get to point approximately 1 km from deli, picture deli in mind and think 'chocolate' > pull into deli > buy chocolate > eat chocolate on remaining journey home. Rebecca would very briefly get the feeling of holding the steering wheel, her foot on the pedals, picturing the deli while standing on the 'S'.
- *Mandy:* Bath children > feed children > put children to bed > clear away dinner things > tidy toys > sit on sofa > pick up remote and turn on television > feel 'collapsed/bored' and think 'food' > go to refrigerator or pantry and get food > come back and sit on lounge and eat while watching television. Mandy would stand on the 'S' and briefly imagine herself collapsed on the sofa with the television on.
- *Jack:* Arrive home from work > greet spouse > spouse mentions name of relative > feel 'tight in chest' and think 'beer' > go to refrigerator and get beer. Jack would stand on the 'S' and see the relative's face in front of him, or mentally hear his wife saying their name.
- *Peta:* Working at desk in afternoon, look at clock > become aware of fatigue and think 'Mars Bar' > go to confectionery machine and purchase Mars Bar > eat chocolate bar at desk. Peta would stand on the 'S' and imagine herself sitting at her desk and thinking of the confectionery machine, or she would imagine sitting at her desk and looking at the clock.

If we 'take out' any part of the chain of responses at or prior to the feeling that precedes the movement towards the food, we will 'ruin the recipe' and alter the unconscious behavioural strategy that leads to non-hungry eating.

IT'S NOT JUST FOR FOOD!

The resource triangle can be used to treat any negative feelings or beliefs. Take another look at Part 1 to get some ideas of the types of emotional factors that could be preventing you from eating well or exercising enough. If you have any negative emotions or beliefs, definitely treat them with the resource triangle!

So, when you run the resource triangle on problem thoughts or feelings, what type of results can you expect? Look what happened for

CHAPTER 7 EMOTIONAL TRIGGERS TO EATING

Maria and Jo below, and you'll see that often the results can seem magical. When you eliminate the old, troublesome feeling, you automatically start to behave in ways that support health and wellbeing.

Maria didn't try to debate whether or not she had time for sport, or whether or not she should feel guilty. She didn't judge her thoughts or feelings—she just treated them! Likewise, Jo didn't try to force herself to eat better. She just became aware of the thoughts and feelings that preceded unhelpful eating and treated them.

Case studies

Case 3: Maria was too busy to play sport

Maria enjoyed playing tennis when she was younger but she had not played for many years. Indeed, she did not exercise at all. Maria's reasons for not exercising were varied:

- guilt over taking time for herself
- guilt that she would be 'playing' instead of working
- a belief that she didn't have the time or the energy.

Maria successfully used the resource triangle to treat both her guilt and the belief that she just didn't have the time or energy. The result was that Maria began to feel a strong interest and excitement about playing tennis. Her 'reasons' for not playing seemed to disappear into thin air and she found herself playing tennis not just once a week but five times a week! She didn't have to *try* to fit it in—it just seemed to happen.

Maria reported that her energy levels and sense of wellbeing increased dramatically and she found it hard to understand why she had waited so long.

As an added benefit, Maria used NLP techniques to improve her game!

Case 4: Jo loved eating dinner in front of the television

Jo worked quite long hours and when she got home she would grab a processed meal and collapse in front of the television.

She said she was too exhausted to cook and just needed to veg out. After she'd eaten she felt even more tired and would go to bed, waking the next day feeling heavy and low in energy.

Realising that something had to be done, Jo used the resource triangle to treat the feelings 'I'm too tired to cook' and 'I feel like crying if I can't eat in front of the television' and continued her habit.

She repeated this each evening and shortly made the decision to whip up a salad and enjoy it in style at the dining table. To her surprise, she found she stayed up later enjoying a favourite show, yet woke the next morning feeling more refreshed.

Notice that in both cases these people did not use willpower or positive thinking to try to force changes. They simply treated their 'triggers' and found that change then occurred naturally.

However, if they had not had the commitment to treat the problem triggers, then of course nothing would have changed! You don't need willpower to change your eating or exercising behaviour, but you do need willpower to use these powerful tools in order to enjoy such effortless and permanent changes!

Chapter 8
The autopilot that lives your life for you: your self-image

There are thousands of pieces of programming inside your head that run automatically. Collectively, these form the autopilot that runs your life when you're not looking. Like any autopilot, it follows a set of rules, or programming, that respond to feedback in order to stay on its designated track. If the programming contains an error, the autopilot won't recognise the error—it will just keep on flying right into whatever lies ahead, because it doesn't think for itself.

This chapter will help you to:

✓ Find out how your 'identity' or your beliefs about yourself determine your attitudes and behaviours.

✓ Use NLP logical levels to better understand the role of identity and as a tool for automatic change.

✓ Use the amazing Be Set Free Fast technique, probably the fastest method ever devised to rapidly remove blocks to confidence and self-esteem.

PART 2 TECHNIQUES FOR EFFORTLESS CHANGE

Your self-image (identity) as autopilot

How can you consistently behave any differently from what you believe about yourself? You cannot. Can you speak confidently in front of others if deep down you believe yourself to be inferior? Can you choose to regard yourself as an athlete if your deep beliefs say that being an athlete requires certain criteria that you do not meet?

Probably the most important work you can do to promote change involves changing your self-image or identity. And I don't just mean changing your hairstyle or moving the furniture! When you make changes to your environment, you don't necessarily change who or what you think you are. But when you change your self-image or identity, everything changes.

LOGICAL LEVELS

'Logical levels' refer to the model of 'neurological levels' originated by anthropologist Gregory Bateson and developed by Robert Dilts. These are shown in Figure 8.1. In this hierarchy of levels of thinking, the higher levels 'rule over' the levels below. If you change something at one of the lower levels, it doesn't necessarily change that something all the way up the hierarchy. However, if you change something at one of the higher levels, it causes changes in every level below. This is why making a change at the level of identity tends to have a domino effect on all the levels below, whereas merely changing something in your environment may have very little effect at all.

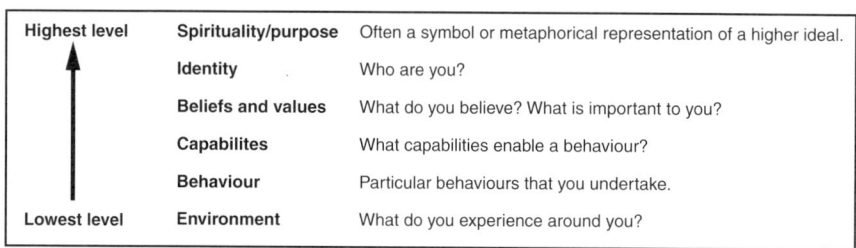

Figure 8.1 Logical levels

You can use logical levels to solve problems, set goals or achieve more congruency in the way you live.

EXERCISE

Imagine the feeling of being effortlessly slim, including having fantastic health and wellbeing. Imagine being like this, including the context in which you would like to experience it.

1. As a floor exercise, step out the various logical levels by actually walking one step forward for each level, commencing with the environment level and ending with the spiritual/purpose level. As you step into each level, describe out loud the significance of the level to the state of being effortlessly slim.

   For example, at the environment level, describe a place where you want to experience being effortlessly slim and healthy (it doesn't matter which place you choose, just select a typical environment for you); at the behaviour level, describe the ways in which your behaviour (your actions) supports being effortlessly slim and healthy; at the capability level, describe the skills and knowledge you have that allow you to engage in the actions/behaviour that support your slimness and health; at the beliefs and values level, describe what you believe that allows you to use these skills and knowledge; at the identity level, describe who you are to have these beliefs; and at spirituality/purpose level, describe your overall purpose or vision for your life (perhaps as a symbol).

   Notice how your vision of your purpose affects every other level.

   To follow is an example of what someone might describe as they move from one level to the next:

   - *Environment level:* I see my kitchen and the bench top in front of me. My children are sitting on the other side and I hear them telling me about their day at school. I smell the food I'm preparing. I feel the knife in one hand and the smooth edge of the watermelon in the other (notice I'm using several senses here).
   - *Behaviour level:* I'm standing up, slicing into the watermelon, some orange and banana and putting this

on a plate in front of my children. We eat it together, and I notice how really delicious this is. I feel real pleasure.
- *Capabilities level:* I understand the importance of fruit in my children's diet (and mine) and I have the ability to choose healthy food for my family. I enjoy learning new things and am willing to make changes if I discover that I've been in error. I'm aware that I have a quality of determination that my children are learning to recognise and I enjoy healthy eating.
- *Beliefs and values level:* I believe that every child has the right to grow up healthy, and to get proper nutrition and physical exercise. It's important to me to be a great role model for my children. It's also important to me to have the best life that I can, and I know this depends on treating my body well. I really value quality of life for my family and it's important for me to embrace all that this entails.
- *Identity level:* I am a woman, a mother, a wife, a teacher, a friend, a daughter, a sister and an aunt. I am a tennis player. 'Truth' is important to me, insofar as I can discern it.
- *Spirituality/purpose level*: I have a feeling that could be described in some ways as 'sacred' and I sense my connection with everything as if I were a drop of water in a vast ocean. In fact, it is the ocean that symbolises this level for me. The 'ocean' is 'love'.

2. Maintaining this clarity of vision/purpose, step back into the identity level and feel your identity merge with your purpose.
3. Maintaining your purpose and identity, step back into the beliefs and values level and feel them all merge.
4. Continue stepping back into each level, bringing the merged qualities of the other levels with you, until you are back at the environment level, knowing that you have all these resources at your fingertips, perfectly aligned and congruent, whenever you wish to use them.

CHAPTER 8 YOUR SELF-IMAGE

The role of your subconscious mind

Your subconscious mind is not only your 'autopilot', it is also your 'obedient servant'. It appears to exist in order to fulfil two purposes: to ensure your physical survival and wellbeing; and to carry out explicit orders or commands.

Your subconscious mind effortlessly and faultlessly carries out many thousands of activities simultaneously at any given time. It has the capacity to control *every single individual muscle fibre in your body*. It runs unimaginably complex chemical and mechanical processes 24 hours a day. It is *always* seeking instruction and it always does what it is told, providing some simple rules are followed.

Knowing how to communicate effectively with your subconscious mind is both a science and an art—BSFF takes care of both!

In the following text, I use the terms 'unconscious mind' and 'subconscious mind'. They mean the same thing: the part of your neurological processing that is outside of your conscious awareness. Don't get hung up on which term is correct, like some people do. The world's most elite psychiatrists can't agree on it, so you certainly shouldn't stress out over it!

What is BSFF?

BSFF was developed by clinical psychologist Dr Larry Phillip Nims and is a system of treatment that effectively eliminates the unconscious, automatic responses that comprise problem feelings, attitudes, beliefs and behaviours. BSFF asserts that the unconscious mind has the capacity to eliminate these responses because it created them in the first place. BSFF maintains that it certainly will eliminate these behaviours because it is very amenable to our commands, provided we understand how to command it accurately and precisely.

In other words, BSFF 'undoes' or extinguishes unconscious programming. Obviously, this has many uses, and one of the uses where BSFF shines is in its application to self-image.

The role of muscle testing

Muscle testing involves the use of ideomotor (subconscious movement) responses to determine the true/false agreement of the subconscious

63

mind with statements we make. To illustrate how the subconscious mind controls muscle strength, try this simple lifting exercise, being careful to protect your back.

Exercise

Stand behind a chair, bracing yourself well with your feet shoulder-width apart. Grasp the chair ready to lift it. Say 'My name is …' (giving your correct name) and then lift the chair a very short distance in the air and put it down. Next, say 'My name is …' (using a false name) and again lift the chair a very short distance in the air and put it down. Most people report the chair feeling 'heavier' the second time—this is because muscle strength is reduced with a false statement.

Your muscles generally cannot lock with the same strength when you make a statement that your subconscious mind believes to be incorrect.

You can also try using these statements:

- *I am sitting down (if it's true).*
- *I am standing up (if it's false).*
- *I am wearing a blue cardigan (if it's true).*
- *I am wearing a pink tutu (if it's false).*
- *2 + 2 is 4.*
- *2 + 2 is 5.*

So, a 'strong' muscle lock is evidence of agreement with a statement, and a 'weak' muscle lock is evidence of disagreement with a statement ('true' and 'false' responses). Each of us is a walking lie detector!

A small percentage of people will get inconsistent or unhelpful results. In such cases, it may be helpful to visit a kinesiologist or to work with a qualified hypnotherapist to develop a more reliable ideomotor signal set-up. (Pendulum movement is mediated by the same psycho-cybernetic response and may also be used.)

Thus, muscle testing is an important (though not foolproof) window into the subconscious. You cannot otherwise know with any certainty what the subconscious contains—or it wouldn't be subconscious! People are often surprised to find that subconscious beliefs directly contradict what they consciously believe. By using muscle testing, you can determine what lies at the root of a problem, and also what progress you are making.

You need to practise muscle testing to reach a degree of proficiency, and you must always be alert to the possibility of influencing the result. (See 'Trouble-Shooting Muscle Testing' in the manual *Unlimited Confidence and Charisma* by The Lifeworks Group for a discussion on procedures.)

Of course, you don't want to be lifting a chair continuously in order to determine the beliefs of your own subconscious. There are some simple self-testing procedures that can be used. For instance, you can keep a 2 L bottle handy and check the perceived change in its weight. Keep in mind that muscle testing is a skill that requires an objective attitude, and most people require practice in order to start getting results that they are happy with.

Setting up BSFF and confirming its acceptance by your subconscious mind

This is the method you use to get your unconscious mind to undo any mental 'programming' that you wish. Once 'set up', every time you give the command to do so, your unconscious mind will immediately eliminate all negative programming around any problem.

First read through the set-up exercise that follows and then actually do it. After that, all you ever need do is to become aware of a problem and then command your unconscious mind to treat it.

Exercise

1. Decide upon your command word.

   Choose a word or term that will serve as your command to your own unconscious mind to eliminate every single problem that you may ever wish to treat. Some people choose computer terms like 'delete' or 'clear', some like to choose spiritual words, and others have fun with words or phrases like 'sticky date pudding'. The meaning of the word or term may be important for your conscious mind, but it is absolutely meaningless to your unconscious mind except as a trigger to eliminate the entire array of unconscious responses that underpin a problem. The words 'death and destruction' would serve just as well!

2. Command your subconscious mind what to do.

   Tell your subconscious mind that whenever you issue the command word, it will immediately go in and eliminate every single emotional root and deepest cause of any problem you may ever wish to treat. And it will do this in such a way that nothing could ever make you want to keep it or take it back, or passively or actively receive it back, or be receptive or vulnerable to it coming back, ever, in any way, shape or form. In addition, it will treat the problem all the way back through your life, through your birth, through your time in the womb and even before. It will continue treating the problem every second of every minute of every hour until you tell it otherwise.

3. Muscle test to confirm your subconscious mind's acceptance of the command.

   You now need to muscle test the following statements:

   (a) *I believe that I can use this simple technique to eliminate any problem I may ever wish to treat.*

   About 50 per cent of people test 'weak' to this statement and will need correction. To correct, just tell your subconscious mind to treat whatever is in the way of accepting this belief and use your new command word. With retesting of the statement, you should test 'strong'. If this is not the case, help will be required.

   There are some simple things you can do to 'fix' muscle testing so that it 'works' properly. For example:

   - have a drink of water
   - move to another room
   - go outdoors
   - turn around 180°
   - remove all metal jewellery

CHAPTER 8 YOUR SELF-IMAGE

- tell your unconscious mind 'Lock my arm very strongly for "true" and make it very weak for "false"'.

In the unlikely event that these simple interventions don't get the results you want, you may need to visit a kinesiologist to get extra help.

(b) *My subconscious mind will do this for me.*

This statement has never been known to test weak, providing of course that statement (a) has been dealt with.

In order to use the BSFF technique now and in the future, you need to have a focus for the treatment and then say the command 'Subconscious mind, treat that, ★ [command word]'. It is important that you make this a *command* and do not say 'Please treat that, ★' or 'Would you now treat that, ★'. These are queries, not commands, and the subconscious mind does not have the ability to respond adequately to anything other than a command.

4. Apply BSFF to your problems.

You are now ready to treat any problem of which you are aware using the statement 'Subconscious mind, treat that, ★ [command word]'. It is not necessary to verbalise the problem—you only need to notice that something is not as you wish and direct the treatment at that 'something'.

Although you can now commence treatment of any issue, it is highly recommended that self-esteem issues are your starting point. These can be dealt with exceedingly quickly and will add to the ease of treating other issues.

Be thorough! On pages 69–71 you will find a list of statements that you should muscle test to determine their truth or fallacy. Keep in mind that you are not testing your logical, conscious beliefs. You are testing your subconscious mind, because this is where the problems are located and this is the part of you that mediates muscle testing.

5. Challenge your results!

BSFF is a powerful, reliable intervention. It is not necessary to 'convince' yourself of its effectiveness, and the apparent

67

changes that you've made are not fragile and do not need to be handled with kid gloves! Rather, in order to be thorough and to be sure that you have done your job, you need to strongly challenge the results.

Muscle testing while you make various statements and/or while you imagine various scenarios involving the problem(s) is a good way to challenge your results. Challenge for past, present and future.

You may not actually feel better (see 'Generalised Anxiety' in the manual *Unlimited Confidence and Charisma* by The Lifeworks Group), but you should certainly expect to see solid and lasting changes in your life immediately and permanently following treatment.

You also need to be aware that other issues may surface now as you go about your life. These are to be welcomed as additional aspects that also require treatment.

USING BSFF FOR IMPROVED SELF-IMAGE

Self-confidence and self-esteem issues are at the heart of many problems. Sooner or later, whether you want to or not, you will be faced with the need to deal with these core issues. To follow is a list of statements you can test. Notice that in this list there is a mixture of positive and negative statements. This may result in some confusion as you consider which 'should' test strong and which 'should' test weak. This confusion is very handy because it gets the conscious mind out of the way and lowers the risk of interference in the result.

EXERCISE

Work your way through the following statements. Whenever you get a result that is unwanted (e.g. testing weak for 'I like myself'), simply say 'Subconscious mind, treat that, ★ [command word]'. When you retest, the statement should test strong. If it doesn't, repeat the treatment.

If the last statement tests strong, you will need to discover how many other problems are lowering your self-confidence

CHAPTER 8 YOUR SELF-IMAGE

by testing 'There is more than one problem that lowers my self-confidence' and so on, until you get the exact number.

Once this is done, test 'I can treat all these problems together with one treatment of BSFF'. If this tests strong, go ahead and treat, then retest 'There is now no other problem that lowers my self-confidence'.

If muscle testing reveals that all the remaining problems cannot be treated together, merely proceed with 'Subconscious mind, the first problem that lowers my self-confidence, treat that, ★ [command word]; the second problem that lowers my self-confidence, treat that, ★ [command word]' and so on. Again, retest to ensure that none remain.

When I explain this to most people, they gasp with disbelief. 'You mean, I don't even have to know what my problems are?!' I can hardly contain my delight at this realisation. This is exactly right. You don't even need to know what the problem is!

There are more advanced ways to use BSFF if progress seems slow and I very much recommend that if you like this treatment method, you obtain a copy of the manual *Unlimited Confidence and Charisma* by The Lifeworks Group to help build expertise in its use.

STATEMENTS TO CHECK SELF-IMAGE/SELF-CONFIDENCE

- *I like myself.*
- *I'm a good person.*
- *I have personal value and worth.*
- *I deserve good things in life.*
- *I deserve to be loved.*
- *I deserve God's love.*
- *I have a good mind.*
- *I have a good body.*
- *I want to live.*
- *I want to be happy.*
- *I am good at things.*
- *I am a capable person.*
- *I can learn to do almost anything and do it well.*
- *I have a skilful mind.*
- *I have a skilful body.*

PART 2 TECHNIQUES FOR EFFORTLESS CHANGE

- *My body is attractive.*
- *I run my life well.*
- *I want to be successful.*
- *I'm willing to be successful.*
- *I'm willing to be successful now.*
- *I'm willing to do everything necessary to see to it that I'm successful now.*
- *I want to be well.*
- *I'm willing to be well.*
- *I'm willing to be well now.*
- *I'm willing to do everything necessary to see to it that I'm well now.*
- *I'm willing to be happy.*
- *I'm willing to be happy now.*
- *I'm willing to do everything necessary to see to it that I'm happy now.*
- *I get well quickly.*
- *I am confident.*
- *I need to be in control.*
- *I need to excel.*
- *I need to be perfect.*
- *I need to learn/know a lot in order to be happy.*
- *I have love pain.*
- *I have fear of love pain.*
- *I welcome love in my life.*
- *I am responsible for others.*
- *It's not OK for me to have things when others don't.*
- *It's not right for me to have more than others.*
- *If others are struggling, then I must struggle too.*
- *It's OK for me to earn more than ___ a year.*
- *Life is too hard.*
- *I care a lot about what others think of me.*
- *It's OK to express my thoughts.*
- *It's OK to express my feelings.*
- *I have a problem with God.*
- *I have a problem with the Devil.*
- *I have a problem with Hell.*
- *I have a problem with Mum or Dad.*

CHAPTER 8 YOUR SELF-IMAGE

- *I have a problem with a family member.*
- *I have a problem with teachers.*
- *My opinion matters.*
- *I deserve to be listened to.*
- *I deserve time for myself.*
- *I can say 'no' to others with great ease.*
- *I am beautiful inside and out.*
- *I am a superb athlete.*
- *I have a very clever mind.*
- *I am someone who can be admired.*
- *It is perfectly OK for me to stick to my principles.*
- *I fear public speaking.*
- *I have the right to speak.*
- *It's OK to be the centre of attention.*
- *I'm afraid I won't know what to say.*
- *I'm afraid what I say won't come out right.*
- *I don't like people's eyes looking at me.*
- *I believe people are judging me harshly.*
- *I believe people don't like me.*
- *I can't cope if people don't like me.*
- *I believe everyone* must *like me.*
- *I deserve to be fat.*
- *I deserve to be slim.*
- *It's safe for me to be slim.*
- *I won't be a nice person if I'm slim.*
- *I still have at least one problem that lowers my self-confidence.*

Chapter 9
Thinking like a slim person

NATURALLY SLIM PEOPLE generally don't spend their lives thinking about food or about what they should or shouldn't eat. When they do think about food, they use automatic, unconscious strategies that ensure they make the best choices for their health and wellbeing.

This chapter will help you to:

✓ Use an NLP modelling technique to get inside a slim person's head.

CHAPTER 9 THINKING LIKE A SLIM PERSON

Time to Get Fussy About Food!

When you no longer have obsessions and compulsions about food or about eating, you tend to get fussier about the types of foods and beverages you're willing to put in your mouth! When I ask slim people how they decide when and what they eat, an interesting pattern emerges.

This may sound crazy to you, but slim people very often go through a process of *imagining* eating the food they are considering eating. Only when they mentally experience the taste, the way it feels in their mouth, the way it goes down their food pipe, the way it feels in their stomach and perhaps even the effect on their body, do they actually decide whether or not to consume the food. A slim person, hungry and faced with a full refrigerator or pantry, may 'taste' many items or combinations of items before actually deciding what to eat. And, if not overly hungry, a slim person will often simply close the refrigerator or pantry door without selecting anything if nothing 'tastes' too inspiring!

Try this next time you feel hungry. How does it alter the way you think about food?

Getting Inside a Slim Person's Head

One way to comprehensively take on the attitudes and behaviours of a slim person is to use an NLP modelling technique. There are several, and the one I'm about to describe to you is extremely easy! Slimness is a behavioural strategy and behavioural strategies run automatically only when they're underpinned by an internal state (emotion) that provides the 'energy' for the strategy to run. If you wish to model, or copy, a slim person, you need to also experience the internal states that generate the slim person's behavioural sequence, otherwise too much conscious attention will be required to run the strategy.

Exercise

To model a slim person, pick someone to 'model' who exhibits effortless slimness. This person should remain healthy and slim without dieting or thinking about food excessively. You do not need to like everything about this person—you are modelling selectively!

PART 2 TECHNIQUES FOR EFFORTLESS CHANGE

1. Get comfortable in a chair and allow yourself to relax into a really peaceful state.
2. Imagine that you are observing your 'model'. They will not necessarily be engaging in any particular behaviour, but simply going about their life.
3. Imagine that you have a very deep and authentic connection or bond with this person. Do this until you experience a feeling of comfort and trust about being in this person's presence.
4. Mentally step into your model's body and allow yourself to feel their physical movements and internal state(s). How do you need to hold your body now? What is your breathing like? What do you actually feel, physically and emotionally? Is this comfortable? Practise being your model until it feels quite comfortable and quite automatic. Don't concern yourself with the detail, but simply with 'the big picture'.
5. 'Take over' your model until it is not them standing there, but you. Check your posture, breathing and feelings so that they remain as before. Practise being in this state until you feel very comfortable and the process occurs automatically.
6. Step aside from your body and observe yourself easily and naturally exhibiting the behaviour you have just practised so thoroughly.

Chapter 10
Dealing with negative feelings: Emotional Freedom Techniques

I N 1998, news got out on the NLP chat lists about a new therapy called EFT, which claimed results bordering on the miraculous. This new therapy partly involved tapping on energy meridian points. My chat groups went into a sort of frenzy about it, to the point where EFT took over the topic of discussion to the exclusion of the original 'purpose' of the groups. The topic was even banned on some chat lists, and various groups split off to continue uninterrupted discussion and investigation of this seemingly miraculous new approach.

This chapter will help you to:

- ✓ Appreciate EFT as a true neuro-somatic therapy, engaging the body via the autonomic nervous system and neurological processing, simultaneously.
- ✓ Use EFT to collapse or eliminate just about any negative emotion you can think of.

PART 2 TECHNIQUES FOR EFFORTLESS CHANGE

A BRIEF HISTORY OF EFT

> Tapping on the energy system while being tuned into an emotional (or physical) problem is an extraordinary healing technique that is deserving of the Nobel Prize. Its impact on the healing sciences is bound to be enormous (Gallo 1999).

EFT actually has its genesis in traditional Chinese medicine. The ancient Chinese, along with many other ancient cultures, believed that we all have an 'energy body' and that energy flows through this body along lines called 'meridians'. They believed that 'blockages' in the meridians caused illness. They identified many different points on the physical body that, when stimulated, seemed to impact on the energy body and thus influence health. Modern acupuncture and acupressure, as well as reflexology and other energy therapies, have their genesis in traditional Chinese medicine.

You might be surprised to hear that Western science may have finally caught up with this ancient knowledge. Not only can we easily measure changes in electrical resistance at acupuncture points, but in the mid-1980s French researchers provided evidence for the existence of the meridian system. French scientist Pierre de Vernejoul set about testing for the existence of a previously 'unknown' circulatory system by injecting a radioactive tracer dye into acupuncture points. The resulting pattern of dye clearly showed the traditional meridian lines. When the dye was injected into non-acupuncture points, no lines appeared. The lines did not correspond with any circulatory system previously known to science, but nevertheless were physical channels through tissue and organs.

The most important contribution of Western science has been the discovery that when we combine emotional/mental work with stimulation of meridian points, the body and mind appear to work together to gently but quickly eliminate many psychological and physical problems. The whole of our body-mind tends towards health and wholeness ... given appropriate conditions. We know that this is true because time and time again we witness our body and mind repair themselves. We know this is true because when we are born we arrive with 'hard-wired' programming that ensures we eat just the right amount and that we love to move! As we experience various life events,

CHAPTER 10 DEALING WITH NEGATIVE FEELINGS

other 'programming' gets written over the top of our original programming. What we have discovered is that when we eliminate this newer programming, the old 'hard-wired' programming is free to run again—and does!

The first dramatic breakthrough was made by Dr Roger Callahan, who developed thought field therapy (originally called the Callahan techniques), which is a system of diagnosis and treatment of emotional causes according to a range of particular algorithms, or sequences of tapping on precise meridian points.

The story goes that Dr Callahan was working with a chronically phobic patient, Mary, who had such a fear of water that she had to be accompanied by someone wherever she went, just in case she saw so much as a photograph of water. Mary couldn't even face an inch of water in her bathtub, nor could she look at a puddle of water on the road. Dr Callahan deduced that Mary had a blockage in a meridian point just below the eye. Upon tapping this point, Mary's phobia was completely and permanently eliminated and to this day (nearly 20 years later) Mary has no problem with water.

Needless to say, Dr Callahan was extremely excited by his discovery and at first thought he had discovered the cure to all phobias (a sort of therapeutic 'Eureka!' experience). Indeed, some of his clients got results in this way, but others required different or more complex treatment. Eventually, Dr Callahan developed the very complex and sophisticated system known as thought field therapy. This system was structured around the basic principle that there is one, and only one, sequence of tapping points (called an 'algorithm') that can relieve a particular problem. People required a great deal of time and a very large amount of money ($US100 000) to learn the full techniques.

Dr Callahan suffered disdain and ridicule from his own profession as a result of his work and his efforts to bring it to a wider audience. His licence and livelihood were threatened by the governing Psychological Board in California and he was unable to have his excellent research published because no editor would touch this *formerly* highly-esteemed researcher.

I am reminded of that wonderful piece from Ayn Rand's book, *The Fountainhead*:

> Throughout the centuries there were men who took the first steps down new roads armed with nothing but their own vision. Their

goals differed, but they all had this in common: that the step was first, the road new, the vision unborrowed, and the response they received—hatred. The great creators—the thinkers, the artists, the scientists, the inventors—stood alone against the men of their time. Every great new thought was opposed. Every great new invention was denounced. They fought, they suffered and they paid. But they won (Rand 1976).

Since then, NLP Master Practitioner Gary Craig, who was the first person to pay the $US100 000 fee to Dr Callahan to learn his techniques, has discovered that the sequence of tapping is unnecessary. As a trained engineer and a very skilled NLPer, Gary Craig was able to take what he had learned from Callahan and dyna-charge it with NLP principles and techniques.

I am highly suspect of EFT as an 'energy' therapy because I see no evidence of 'energy' being involved, and the research I referred to above has not been replicated successfully. Even the Chinese, who run thousands of pieces of high-quality research every year investigating acupuncture, have not demonstrated the existence of any energy system.

We do know that the acupoints are associated with, or paralleled by, the autonomic nervous system and that tapping them has a direct impact on the brain, particularly the amygdala, which mediates emotional responses. This much has been successfully demonstrated using brain imaging techniques.

So I think of EFT as an application of NLP that incorporates stimulation over the autonomic nervous system (tapping on acupoints) with clever language patterns. When we trigger a negative internal state (a feeling) at the same time that we paradoxically stimulate the brain and nervous system, we appear to actually eliminate this state as an automatic response.

I strongly suspect that the old, conditioned response collapses because of the twin 'interference' patterns run over the top of it. In my upcoming book on treating chronic pain, I will elaborate on this hypothesis. This means that although the same situation or event may recur, we don't have a knee-jerk negative reaction to it. We remain resourceful and in charge of ourselves—we get to choose our response instead of being on the receiving end of an unwanted response!

CHAPTER 10 DEALING WITH NEGATIVE FEELINGS

THE ACTUAL EFT PROCESS

To use the EFT process, the first thing you must do is construct a sentence whose language both triggers your negative emotional state and presents a paradoxical statement (by paradoxical I mean 'contrary' or 'in opposition'). What we say often sounds very negative because we are describing the problem exactly as it is, in our own language, in order to precisely elicit the negative internal state that has presented us with the 'problem'.

This sentence will generally take the form of 'Even though I have this __ [explain problem], I deeply and profoundly love and accept myself'. This sentence is said three times while tapping or rubbing on an acupoint, which I'll describe shortly.

To give you an idea of the type of wording you might use, let's look at an example. One of my clients had such a severe spider phobia that she couldn't go out at night for fear of walking into a web. After tapping on an acupoint saying 'Even though I have this fear of spiders, I deeply and completely accept myself', and then repeating this process for all other acupoints, she had absolutely no improvement.

So I asked her how she might describe her fear to someone else, to which she answered, 'Oh, I'm scared *shitless* of spiders!' Fantastic! This was just what we needed. So I asked her to tap saying 'Even though I'm scared *shitless* of spiders, I deeply and completely accept myself' and she got instant elimination of the problem.

I've seen this happen many times. If you choose words that don't 'resonate' with you, or that don't accurately describe the way you really think about the problem/issue, the results may not be anything remarkable.

The table on page 80 provides more examples of language patterns that you can use to trigger the emotional state you wish to extinguish.

WHERE DO YOU START TAPPING?

There are at least five points that are commonly used to start off the EFT process, but you need to remember only one of them—*the one that you actually like using the most!* You can change the point you use to start off the process, and in fact I use different points depending on how I feel at the time. Experiment now with the points below and get a feel for where they are and how you like each one.

PART 2 TECHNIQUES FOR EFFORTLESS CHANGE

Examples of language patterns

Sentence beginnings	Sentence endings
Even though I'll miss out, ...	I deeply and profoundly love and accept myself.
Even though I'll starve, ...	I choose to be free.
Even though it's not safe to lose weight, ...	I know deep down I deserve the best in life.
Even though it's all too hard, ...	I choose to laugh out loud.
Even though it's bad to waste food, ...	I claim my right to perfect health.
Even though I'm bad if I waste food, ...	Deep down, I know my partner only wants the best for me.
Even though my partner said 'You're stacking it on lately', ...	I deeply and profoundly forgive my partner for being such a pig.
Even though this chocolate is the only love I get, ...	I choose to love myself by making better choices for my mind and my body.

Three of the points are tapped and these are the karate chop point, the thymus point and the underarm point (see Figure 10.1).

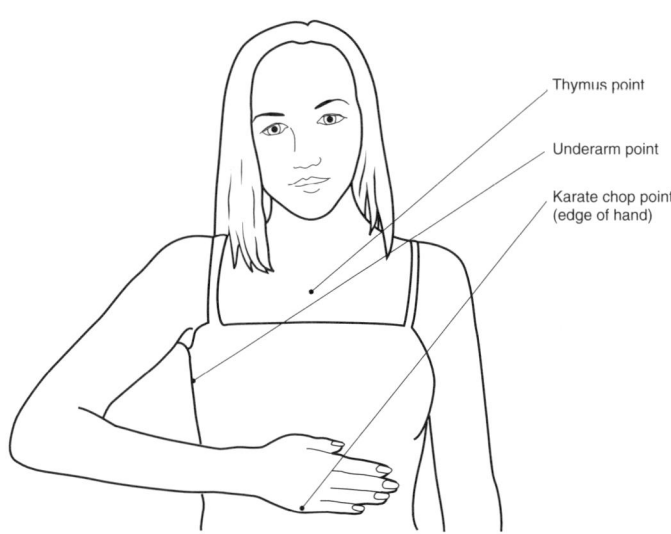

Figure 10.1 Tapping points to use to commence EFT treatment

CHAPTER 10 DEALING WITH NEGATIVE FEELINGS

Two of the points are rubbed and these are the two collarbone points (also known as the K27s), which are rubbed in a circular motion at the same time, usually with one hand, using the thumb and index finger (see Figure 10.2), and the sore spot, which is actually a neurolymphatic reflex point (see Figure 10.3).

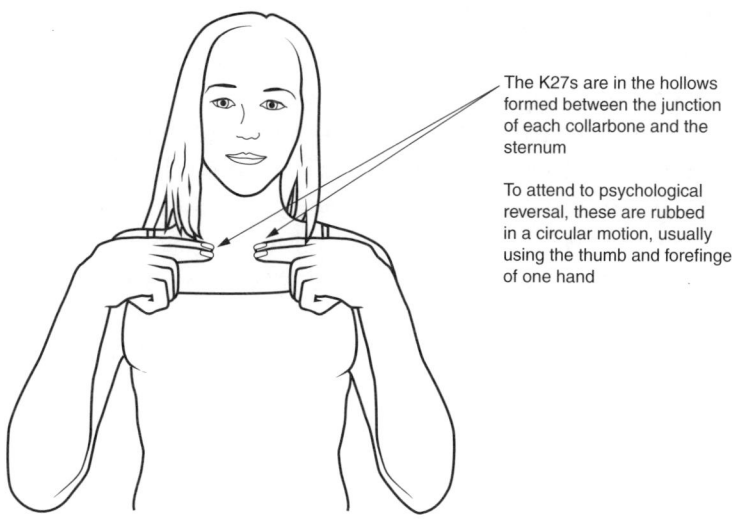

The K27s are in the hollows formed between the junction of each collarbone and the sternum

To attend to psychological reversal, these are rubbed in a circular motion, usually using the thumb and forefinger of one hand

Figure 10.2 Rubbing points to use to commence EFT treatment: the K27s

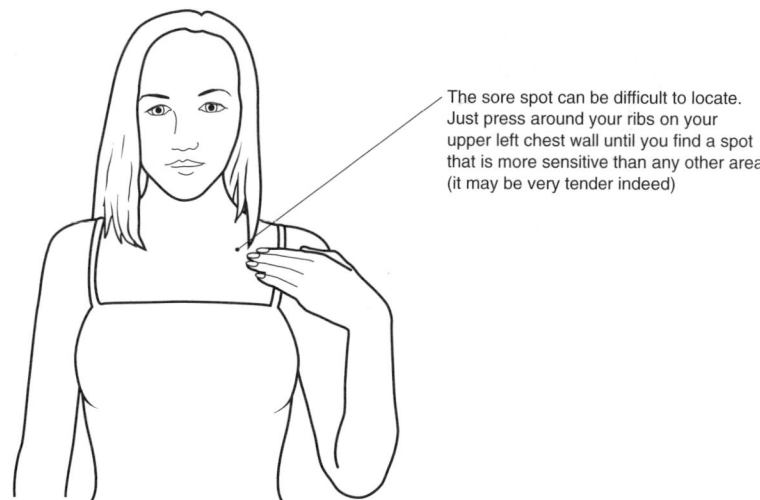

The sore spot can be difficult to locate. Just press around your ribs on your upper left chest wall until you find a spot that is more sensitive than any other area (it may be very tender indeed)

Figure 10.3 An alternative rubbing point to use to commence EFT treatment: the sore spot

In this version of EFT I use nine basic tapping points, which you'll find in Figure 10.4. These points are named very logically as follows: the crown (the top of your head), occipital ridge (the bump on the back of your head), eyebrow (inner edge), outer eye, under eye, top lip, lower lip (actually the chin crease), collarbone (actually just below the collarbone and to one side of the sternum), and underarm (about 7–8 cm down from the armpit).

This series of nine points is used over and over from start to finish as you work through a problem. You might like to tap through them a few times from start to finish just to get the feel of them. I've known people experience surprising results just from doing this! For instance, in one group I was working with, a lady in a wheelchair who was suffering extreme back pain started to 'tap through' with me just to learn the points. She suddenly exclaimed 'My pain's gone!' much to everyone's delighted amazement.

Read the following steps to get a feel for how EFT works. First, you'll need to identify some language that accurately triggers the problem feeling that you wish to eliminate. Perhaps you have some

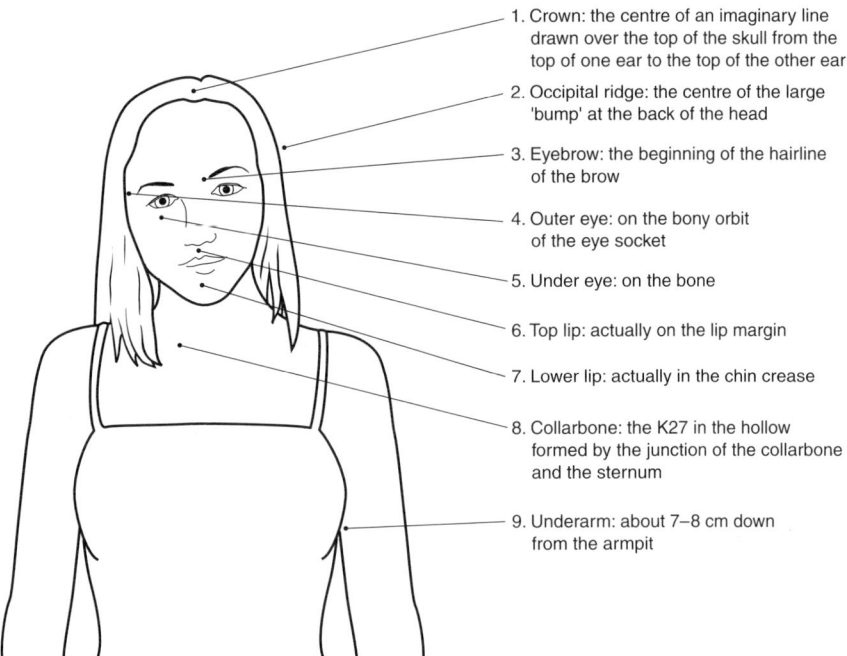

Figure 10.4 The nine tapping points used for EFT 'rounds'

CHAPTER 10 DEALING WITH NEGATIVE FEELINGS

mild anger at someone and would like to get rid of it once and for all, or a craving for chocolate, or are feeling a little tired?

Then give the problem feeling a 'rating' out of 10 to subjectively measure how serious the problem is for you. A score of 10 out of 10 means you can't imagine feeling any more intensity than you do right now and a score of 0 out of 10 means you don't have the feeling at all. *Warning!* Do not choose a problem that rates higher than 5 out of 10 for you! When you've developed both competence and confidence in this technique, you can use it with a much wider range of problems.

Once you've run the problem you've identified through the EFT process, you should notice a decrease in the rating of at least 2–3 points on your subjective scale.

EXERCISE

1. Commence the EFT process by verbally describing the problem while simultaneously tapping or rubbing on your selected starting point (see Figures 10.1, 10.2 and 10.3).

    Construct a sentence that both describes the problem and offers a contrary or opposing statement, and say that sentence three times while tapping or rubbing on one of the five starting points described above.

    The contrary statement doesn't have to relate to the problem part of the sentence at all. If you can make the contrary part humorous, all the better. For example, one client hated going to the beach because he said, with emotion, 'I feel like a beached whale!'. His sentence was: 'Even though I feel like a beached whale, I choose to free Willy!' This worked marvellously well!

2. Tap through the 'rounds' (a series of nine points).

    It is now time to address the nine points that make up the rest of the EFT process. It will take about 10–12 seconds to complete an entire round, perhaps less, and involves tapping 5–7 times on each of the points.

    You also need to *say something* to help maintain your problem state (feeling). This is where you put your whole problem in a nutshell and say a few words (e.g. 'this beached whale feeling') from your initial sentence that serve to represent the whole shebang. Say these words just once for each of the nine points, from your crown down to your underarm.

Repeat the 'round' three times.

3. After three 'rounds' of tapping from crown to underarm, go back and do the initial sentence and starting point again, but say the sentence only once this time. Then tap three rounds of all nine points, saying a few words to keep your problem state. Check how you feel about the problem now. Would you put the same intensity on your feeling or has it diminished?

Now that you've had a 'run through' with EFT and are beginning to gain some confidence using it, let's treat something else. Think of a particular food that you have trouble saying 'no' to. As you think about this food, what words come into your head? For example:

- *Yum, I'd really like that now.*
- *I really, really want that chocolate now.*
- *I just love salty potato chips.*

Take a moment to think how strongly you have this feeling on a scale of 0 to 10.

Now construct your EFT sentence about that food. For example:

- *Even though I really, really want that chocolate right now, I deeply and profoundly love and accept myself.*
- *Even though I really, really want that chocolate right now, I wonder what's on television tonight.*

Look at the examples opposite if you need more ideas.

Exercise

1. Say the sentence you've constructed three times as you tap or rub on one of the five starting points.
2. Now, saying just a few key words (e.g. 'This chocolate feeling'), tap through the nine points of the EFT round, and then repeat the round twice more. Each time you tap on one of the nine points (tap fairly rapidly 5–7 times on

each point), just say, for example, 'This chocolate feeling' once for each point.
3. Go back to your starting point and say your initial sentence just once. Go through the round three times saying the same few key words. Check how you feel about the food now. Would you put the same intensity on your feeling or has it diminished?
4. Repeat steps 1–3 until there's no intensity at all. This means that when you think about the food you were treating with EFT, there is a feeling of complete disinterest. You may or may not eat it, but certainly there is no craving or desire for it. Truly, you can say that this feeling is now '0 out of 10'!

When EFT seems slow or ineffective

Every now and then you may seem to make no or little progress with EFT. This may be a perception (perhaps there are so many interacting aspects that it's not until you've dealt with a proportion of them that you begin to notice a change) or nothing much in fact may be happening.

For beginners, the problem is usually an incomplete or inadequate set-up, not getting into the issue properly or another very routine matter. For instance, often the problem is stated too 'globally' or generally, and a little playing around with the words will produce a very specific wording that comes with the right 'ring' so that you know it's the one to focus on. Here's an example:

> *Even though I just can't lose weight, I deeply and profoundly accept myself.*

This may be a decent starting point if you can't think of anything more specific, but you'll probably find specific thoughts or images popping into your head as you work through it. For instance:

- *I can't stand the sight of myself in the mirror.*
- *I'll starve if I don't eat that chocolate.*
- *I just want to cry when I think about getting fatter.*
- *I'll scream if I have to count one more kilojoule.*
- *I'm angry that my jeans won't do up.*
- *I'm scared my partner will leave me.*

PART 2 TECHNIQUES FOR EFFORTLESS CHANGE

- *I feel so helpless.*
- *I hate those scales.*
- *That woman in the little bikini is a total bitch.*

Working on these specifics will probably uncover things that are even more specific and that may seem unrelated, particularly childhood memories that you consider to be of minor importance. Trust me, they only *seem* irrelevant.

A WORD ABOUT BEING OVERWHELMED

Sometimes, as you 'contact' an emotional issue, it seems that all hell breaks loose as you experience a virtual 'emotional Vesuvius'. You might become aware that a problem has a much bigger impact on you than you first realised, or you might discover something 'underneath' the problem you are working on that is obviously much, much bigger than the initial problem. Or you might suddenly become overwhelmed by a million thoughts racing around in your head and causing distress.

This can happen even when you are in the care of a psychologist or a psychiatrist who is using these methods (or conventional methods) and who is well aware of the landscape of the particular psyche they are working with, the precautions that they can take to keep their client as safe and comfortable as possible, and the action that needs to be taken should distress nevertheless arise.

It should be obvious that it is therefore unsafe for anyone but a fully trained mental health professional to work with other people's issues in this way—hence the warning at the front of this book.

If you find yourself moving into a highly emotional state while working through this book, please get the appropriate help. To continue working on yourself in this state can be likened to a brain surgeon trying to operate on themselves! This help might come from a friend or family member who can at least listen and provide a shoulder to lean on, or it might be the expert help of an appropriate health professional.

There are two approaches that you might like to keep in mind in the interim while you seek assistance, to help you to get back to a comfortable internal state:

1. Contain the problem—ask your unconscious mind to make a picture of or otherwise come up with a 'container' that can hold your

CHAPTER 10 DEALING WITH NEGATIVE FEELINGS

feelings of being overwhelmed. Place your feelings in the container and seal it well.

2. Thank the overwhelming feelings for showing up and tell them that you will certainly deal with each of them, *but* you can only do that one at a time. Sit down and make a list of everything that comes to mind and rate each one on a scale of 0 to 10 (where 0 represents the feeling being no problem at all and 10 represents the highest distress level you can imagine). Most people can safely start working on their list by picking all the lower numbers first. By the time they get to the things that were rated nine or 10, they can rank them much lower.

TO SUMMARISE

You are a product of your memory and learning, with the majority of your memory and learning out of conscious awareness. In other words, the majority of 'drivers' in your life are *unknown* to you. You have no idea where the majority of feelings that you feel originate from, no idea they are at cause in your life and, rather than 'running your own bus', you are being driven by an unknown driver to an unknown destination.

The key to being able to drive the bus yourself is to eliminate the negative emotions attached to old memories. All of us carry memories that are charged with negative emotion to some degree and that are therefore still at cause in our lives.

Chapter 11
Internal settings: what does your unconscious mind think your ideal 'healthy' weight should be?

O FTEN, YOU CONSCIOUSLY DECIDE that you want something and yet there are unconscious mechanisms that prevent you from getting it. One such problem may be your unconscious mind's belief about what is your 'right' weight.

This chapter will help you to:

✓ Use the metaphor of a 'gauge' to get your unconscious mind to do the work for you.

CHAPTER 11 YOUR IDEAL 'HEALTHY' WEIGHT

What weight does your unconscious mind think you should be?

Patty weighed 87 kg and felt that she was around 20 kg overweight. She very much wanted to lose weight but felt that not only was 'something' preventing it, but also that it was a struggle for her to avoid putting on even more weight. We used muscle testing to get an idea of what might be going on in Patty's subconscious, starting off with the statement:

My perfect, healthy weight is 67 kg.

It wasn't actually surprising that this tested weak. We then went on to test the following statements and got the results shown:

- *My perfect healthy weight is less than 70 kg.* Weak
- *My perfect healthy weight is less than 80 kg.* Weak
- *My perfect healthy weight is less than 90 kg.* Weak
- *My perfect healthy weight is less than 100 kg.* Strong

So Patty had a situation where her subconscious mind believed not only that it wasn't healthy for her to be her ideal weight, but also that she should weigh even more than she did. No wonder Patty had struggled.

There are many tools we could have used to deal with these subconscious beliefs. We chose to use metaphors, selecting GaugeWork, developed by Australian therapist Astra Johnston. GaugeWork is interesting enough, complex enough and powerful enough to fill a book all on its own. However, here I'll describe a very simple way of using it that anyone can learn.

GaugeWork

Are you curious what your own unconscious 'setting' for your weight might be? You can muscle test for this, as I did with Patty, or you can use GaugeWork to 're-set' to what you've already decided is right for you.

Warning! Your subconscious programming around weight is frequently a complex array of values and beliefs. It would be simplistic in the extreme to think that you could 're-set' your internal (subconscious) representation of what 'normal, healthy weight' actually means merely by setting a single gauge. If you persist in trying to achieve this, you will be doing so in the face of a lot of internal resistance. This is slow, clumsy and even disrespectful. In order to be thorough, and to achieve results that are enduring, you need to gently attend to the whole complex array of issues around weight. GaugeWork is merely one of the tools that will help you to attend to your internal programming.

In GaugeWork, you need to imagine a gauge that runs from 0 to 100 per cent. Everyone has a different idea about how this gauge should look. Some people immediately imagine a line that runs from left to right, with '0 per cent' on the left and '100 per cent' on the right, and some sort of 'slider' that moves along the line to show the 'measure'. Other people imagine something that looks more like an old-style car odometer, a digital readout, a jug with levels marked on the side or even a thermometer. Children who have used this concept have been particularly creative. One boy used a visualisation of a boat race. The start line was the 0 per cent mark and the finish line was the 100 per cent mark. When his boat (indicating the percentage measure) reached the finish line, balloons and streamers would shoot up into the sky!

Once you've decided on the appearance of your gauge, you need to give the gauge a name that represents the resolution of a problem, then 'look' to see whereabouts on the gauge the needle, slider, marker or level is sitting. For instance, if you would like to get more pleasure out of eating salads, you might call it the 'I love eating salads' gauge. Now, if you think salads are rabbit food, you will probably notice that your gauge is sitting at perhaps only 10 per cent.

Interestingly, when you direct your unconscious mind to 'set that gauge on 100 per cent' and imagine moving the slider along, pouring liquid into the jug or whatever, you not only notice that it is very easy to imagine, but you also notice a very rapid change in your attitudes and behaviours!

It's not necessary to give your gauge a positive-sounding name. For instance, you could have a gauge called 'No desire whatsoever for junk food'. In fact, as you gain more experience with using gauges, you will find it quite essential to include 'absence of negative' gauges in order to deal thoroughly with a particular problem.

Most people are highly surprised that the gauge 'works'. It really does seem to 'cooperate' with the task at hand—and why not when

CHAPTER 11 YOUR IDEAL 'HEALTHY' WEIGHT

the subconscious operates in the language of metaphors? You are literally 'talking the right language' when you use metaphors to communicate with your subconscious.

If you are thinking 'This won't work for me because I don't see pictures', or if you don't like to make mental pictures or find it too challenging, you can use your hands as the gauge instead. Simply put your hands out in front of you, palms facing one another with perhaps an 80 cm gap in between, and nominate one hand to represent 0 per cent and the other to represent 100 per cent. You can then move the hand that represents 0 per cent towards the hand that represents 100 per cent instead of moving a marker.

The GaugeWork process is as follows:

1. Decide on a problem you want to deal with.
2. Imagine a gauge (whatever type of gauge suits you best).
3. Give the gauge a name that represents the resolution of the problem you wish to deal with.
4. Check where the 'level' of the gauge is. Don't debate with yourself, just forget the name you've given the gauge and merely focus on the gauge itself. If you're using your hands as a gauge, move the hand that represents 0 per cent towards the hand that represents 100 per cent and see where it starts to feel awkward or less smooth. This is your starting level.
5. Now talk to your unconscious mind by commanding it to set this gauge on 100 per cent: 'Unconscious mind, set that gauge on 100 per cent!'
6. In your imagination, move the gauge level to 100 per cent. If you're using your hands as a gauge, move the hand that represents 0 per cent towards the hand that represents 100 per cent. When your hands touch, that represents 100 per cent.

Sometimes the gauge seems to 'stick', meaning that it seems to become stuck at a point below 100 per cent, or that even though it gets to 100 per cent, it keeps coming back. This problem is addressed below.

Exercise

Sit in a comfortable chair and allow yourself time to move into a relaxed and peaceful state. Imagine a mental gauge that runs from 0 to 100 per cent. Let's name this gauge 'My perfect healthy weight is X kg' (fill in the weight). Now let's see how true this is for you, between 0 and 100 per cent. Where on this gauge does the level or needle sit? If you are using your hands, how far along can you comfortably move one hand towards the other?

Most likely your gauge will fall short of the 100 per cent mark. In such a case, simply say to your unconscious mind in a commanding tone of voice 'Set that on 100 per cent and I mean it!' and observe what happens next. For some people, the gauge will go up and stay up. For others, it will go up and slide back somewhat. If this happens, simply repeat the process regularly until one day you check your gauge and find that it stays up at 100 per cent all by itself.

If the gauge 'sticks'

It's not unusual for some gauges to seem to 'stick'. Your slider, gauge needle or level (or however you imagine your gauge) might seem to refuse to move to the 100 per cent mark, or it might go to the 100 per cent mark and then slip back. Here are some things you can experiment with in order to get your gauge to move to the 100 per cent mark and stay there!

1. 'Treat' the gauge with your BSFF command word. To do this, as you notice the gauge appear to stick, or as you get a feeling that it's difficult to move, simply direct your unconscious mind to unblock whatever the problem is by treating it with your BSFF command word. With your attention on the gauge level, and for the moment forgetting all about the name of the gauge, simply say 'Unconscious mind, treat that [command word]'. Remember to use command tonality! Often, this is enough to get the gauge moving smoothly along to the 100 per cent mark.
2. Investigate the gauge more closely. What is stopping the needle from moving? Is there some obstruction? A mechanical problem? Remember that in metaphorland you can call in any resources you wish to get your gauge working. You can take an orbital grinder to it to smooth it off, pour oil or anti-rust on it, and bring in cranes or a whole engineering team—whatever you need to make it work.

CHAPTER 11 YOUR IDEAL 'HEALTHY' WEIGHT

One of my workshop participants reported that her gauge looked like a door runner and that it had grains of sand in it that were preventing the slider from moving along. I asked her what could help and she brought in an imaginary vacuum cleaner. That did the job beautifully!

3. Is there a negative thought that applies to the gauge—for example, 'It's too hard', 'It's not safe' or 'It might work for others but not for me'? In this case, a further gauge or two is called for. You might like to try gauges with these titles:

No reason whatsoever to be hard.
Incredibly easy.
No reason whatsoever to be unsafe.
Absolutely safe.
No reason not to work perfectly for me.
Works perfectly easy for me.

Notice that I've used gauge names that firstly eliminate the negative thought and secondly affirm the positive thought. I call this 'approaching the issue from two directions'. When you return to the original gauge, you'll find it works easily and naturally without a hitch.

USING GAUGES FOR OTHER ISSUES

The things that gauges can be used to treat are limited only by your imagination. For example, one of my clients had a severe snake phobia that he had had since he was scared by a snake when he was eight years old. Now, as an elderly man living in the suburbs, he never went into his own backyard at night for fear a snake might be there.

I constructed one simple gauge for him, 'I love snakes', and worked this in the session until it stayed on 100 per cent. The next week, when he arrived for his second session, I asked how his snake phobia was. He looked quite surprised as he realised that he had completely forgotten about it and had been out in his backyard five times at night in that one week.

Are you angry with someone? Try a gauge for 'No anger at X whatsoever' and see what happens. Would you like more calm, more happiness? Gauge for them!

Part 3
Sabotage: how you stop yourself from getting what you want, and ways to stop the stoppers!

Chapter 12
Identifying your sabotaging thinking and behaviour

IF YOU HAVE STRUGGLED with your weight, you will be familiar with the concept of sabotage. Unfortunately, in the past you've 'worn the blame' for this, unappreciative of the fact that your conscious mind is not 'running the show'. Now you can notice sabotage occurring and treat it, but you should also appreciate some of the unconscious mechanisms that have served to defeat your conscious will.

This chapter will help you to:

✓ Dismiss good reasons for avoiding change.
✓ Appreciate the impact that family and friends can have.
✓ Understand guilt—the Big Kahuna!

PART 3 SABOTAGE

Understanding the consequences of change

When I was struggling with my weight, I tried to imagine what it would be like to be slim and healthy. To my surprise and distress, the only image that would come to mind was of an old sick and starving horse in a paddock, with all its bones sticking out. Being a fan of metaphors, I tried bringing in imaginary vets and trainers and even a playmate, all to no avail. I just couldn't make 'slim' equal 'healthy'.

This is not surprising, especially for a woman. Women are often the nurturers in their families and have been so for generations. Often, when they've experienced a person or a creature in their care as being 'slim', that person or creature may have been about to die. Women have wanted their babies and toddlers to look rounded because they feared for their health. There can be a lot of fear around slimness. Women can have a real difficulty believing that their circumstances are safe and they don't need extra 'stores' just in case things get tough. Slimness can mean an unacceptable vulnerability.

So safety is a big issue—not only concerning a basic fear of starving to death, but also in relation to being safe around the opposite sex. Many people express a belief that they are safer or more relaxed if they are overweight, because then they don't feel so attractive to the opposite sex and don't have to worry about being 'hit on'.

You can see that being overweight may have definite advantages, but these need to be treated if you are to ensure unconscious alignment with a conscious desire to be slim and healthy. BSFF provides a great way to discover and treat the unconscious advantages of being overweight, as well as the unconscious disadvantages of being slim.

Exercise

1. Try muscle testing these statements (fill in the weight):

    - *It's safe for me to be X kg now.*
    - *It's not safe for me to be X kg now.*
    - *I deserve to be X kg now.*
    - *I deserve to be fat now.*
    - *I give myself permission to be X kg now.*
    - *I won't be a nice person if I am X kg.*

CHAPTER 12 YOUR SABOTAGING THINKING AND BEHAVIOUR

If the first sentence tested 'strong', then it doesn't need to be treated because your subconscious believes it to be true. However, if the second sentence tested 'strong', this would represent a problem! If you are working towards a weight that your subconscious believes to be unsafe, you are likely to strike considerable resistance!

2. How many different endings can you give to the following sentences? Be as creative as possible. Don't be concerned about logic or 'truth', just scribble down as many endings as you can. Muscle test each of them to discover what your internal programming is. Which ones should be treated?

- *It's helpful being overweight because* _____.
- *It's helpful being underweight because* _____.
- *It's helpful being slim because* _____.
- *It's unhelpful being overweight because* _____.
- *It's unhelpful being underweight because* _____.
- *It's unhelpful being slim because* _____.

3. How many statements can you construct, test and treat using any of the techniques you've learned so far? You'll probably find these issues amenable to EFT, BSFF, the resource triangle or GaugeWork.

FANTASTICAL THINKING

I love introducing the concept of fantastical thinking in my workshops. It applies to just about all our beliefs! Fantastical thinking involves beliefs such as:

- *When I'm slim I'll go for a better job and earn more money.*
- *When I'm slim I'll travel.*
- *When I'm slim I'll take up dancing.*
- *When I'm slim I'll find a partner who loves me and wants to marry me.*
- *When I'm slim I'll be happy.*

These are all nonsensical of course, because, for most of us, they are all possible whatever weight we might be. I think sometimes we use fantastical thinking as a buffer, as a way of preventing failure by delaying trying. In any case, these beliefs merely serve to delay quality of life because we are declaring that we can't have these things 'until' something happens.

Probably the fastest way to treat these beliefs is to turn them into statements that can be muscle tested and treated using BSFF. For example:

- *I can go for a better job now.*
- *I am willing to go for a better job now.*
- *I am willing to do whatever it takes to go for a better job now.*

THE IMPACT OF YOUR FAMILY AND FRIENDS

Before discussing how to use the meta model to deal with criticism or manipulation (see Chapter 13), let's first look at the people you've gathered around you over the years.

Your family

Although you can't choose your family, you certainly *can* choose how you interact with them. The way they act now is the net result of many, many communication choices you've made over the years, both consciously and unconsciously (without realising it).

At the moment, whether you realise it or not, you have trained your family to help keep you right where you are. If you don't think this is the case, just stand back and watch them as you make changes. Most families go into a game called 'uproar', where they carry out their normal dynamics, but this time louder, or more often.

Virginia Satir, a brilliant and much-loved family therapist, said that families are really dynamic systems. To give people a better idea of how family systems work, she compared the family to a mobile, the type you might hang above a baby's crib. When you take hold of one piece of the mobile and change its position, the rest of the pieces jiggle about madly. Eventually, the other pieces run out of kinetic energy and become still. The important thing to realise is that *they become still in a new position, based on the new position of the one piece that moved.*

In NLP there is a basic supposition that says in part 'The piece of the system with the greatest flexibility is the piece that controls the system'. Families are just like that.

So when you start to make changes in yourself, think of yourself as a piece of that mobile. Now you can understand why your partner might seem crankier than usual, the children might come down with more colds, there are more arguments, or whatever. If you were to ask them, none of them would be able to put their finger on a reason,

CHAPTER 12 YOUR SABOTAGING THINKING AND BEHAVIOUR

although they well might rationalise their behaviour: 'I'm just tired', 'It's not me who's being cranky, it's you' or 'There are a lot of bugs going around'. In fact, they are being driven, unconsciously, to try to put things back where they were.

What I'm talking about here is all quite normal in families. However, for some people, the examples I've given may even seem mild. For example, people in abusive relationships may actually be at real physical risk if they dare to vary their behaviour from the 'norm'. Some relationships are very, very controlling and abusive. One partner will berate and humiliate the other for an inadequacy or 'fault', such as a weight problem, but at the same time will become even more vicious if their partner attempts to do something about it!

It is well and truly beyond the scope of this book to provide adequate support or advice for such people. If you recognise something of this in your relationship, please get expert support to help and guide you through it. You deserve better, and you deserve to be able to make these changes safely.

Your friends

Who you have as friends says an incredible lot about you. What sort of people do you hang out with? Are they similar to you? Are you a 'good news club', or do you spend most of your time together blaming everyone else, sharing woes and commiserating or 'supporting' each other?

Friendship networks are systems too, just like families. So when you make changes you will tend to observe some upset among your friends. They may try harder to sabotage your efforts. They may become critical of you.

It is not only difficult to stay friends with people who cannot grow and support you in the positive, healthy changes you wish to make, it may well be impossible. They will feel a lack of commonality and a lack of connection. Commonly, you won't *have* to leave them because *they* will feel repelled by you in any case.

Therefore, it's important to cultivate new friendships with people who are 'on track' with you. One of the best pieces of advice given to people who want to be successful is to spend time with successful people. If you want a positive, healthy mind-set, spend time with people who have a positive, healthy mind-set.

GUILT: THE BIG KAHUNA!

Guilt is an amazingly efficient saboteur! Many of us, particularly women, experience feelings of guilt or unworthiness when we think about taking time out for our health or wellbeing. There is a tendency to put the needs of everyone else first. The great problem with this attitude of guilt or unworthiness is that not only are we robbing our family and friends of the experience of relating to and being with a fully healthy person, but we are serving as a highly destructive role model to others, particularly children.

Do you really want the world to be a better, kinder place? Do you really want your children growing up knowing how to get healthy and stay healthy? Or would you prefer your children to be just like you, putting themselves last and allowing their health to suffer as a result?

The work that you do now to eliminate guilt over health and 'nurture time' is of vital importance. It cannot be put off, because every day you hesitate is a day where you are demonstrating to others what not to do! Every day you hesitate in getting free of those old burdens is a day going backwards in terms of health and wellbeing.

Remember that getting free of guilt will mean saying 'no' to people as you demonstrate responsible self-care. You are also teaching others how to say 'no' and not all lessons are easy! See Chapter 13 on the meta model for some great retorts to stop criticism or manipulation in its tracks!

Be gentle with those around you who seem to act selfishly or who do not yet appreciate the new, healthier you. Be firm at all times, but keep in mind they may need extra assurance of your love and appreciation for them.

Which technique is best for eliminating guilt relating to taking time out for your health? Probably the resource triangle.

INSTALLING MOTIVATION: THE NLP TIMELINE TECHNIQUE

WALKING THE TIMELINE

Timeline work involves either imagining or marking out on the floor a line that represents the whole of your life. One end represents your birth and the other end stretches out into an infinite future. The timeline is not real. It merely serves as yet another incredibly useful metaphor

CHAPTER 12 YOUR SABOTAGING THINKING AND BEHAVIOUR

and, like the gauges you've been playing with, can be manipulated easily in order to achieve real and lasting change in your life.

EXERCISE

1. Imagine that you have a line stretching out before you that represents the whole of your life. You can imagine this as a mental picture, you can close your eyes and get a 'feel' for where it is, or, if you prefer, you can actually mark it out with chalk or paper on the floor. Whichever option you choose, you are going to be physically walking along your timeline and experiencing your life in different ways.

    The beginning of your timeline is some time before your birth and the ending is somewhere way off in the future. Mark a spot on the timeline that represents the last time you were slim and mark another spot that represents 'now'. Then mark a spot in the future that is equidistant from 'now'— that is, if there is 2 m between the last time you were slim and 'now', this spot will be 2 m into the future.

2. Stand on the spot that represents the last time you were slim, then walk forward to 'now' and look back along the period where you have been overweight and unhealthy.

3. Imagine that 'now' someone gives you the tools that not only will cause you to make permanent changes to ensure you achieve and maintain a slim, healthy body, but that will dramatically enhance your pleasure and quality of life. Imagine further that you make a commitment to using these tools for at least five minutes every day.

4. Now walk forward to the next mark you've made on your timeline knowing that you have used the tools and made the changes and that you are slim and healthy. How does it feel? Be conscious of feeling strong muscles, oxygen moving through your body, energy and a healthy 'glow'.

5. Walk further on into the future and look back over all the time that you've remained slim and healthy. How does it feel? Now walk further into the future, looking out along the timeline and experiencing health and wellbeing. How does it feel?

PART 3 SABOTAGE

6. Step aside from your timeline and try it a different way:

   (a) Stand on the spot that represents the last time you were slim and walk forward to the spot marked 'now', looking back over all the time when you've struggled with your weight and have been so dissatisfied. Notice how this feels.

   (b) Still on the spot marked 'now', imagine that you are offered the tools to make permanent, wonderful changes, but this time you say 'no'.

   (c) Walk forward to the next mark you've made, knowing that nothing has changed and that nothing will change. Looking back over all this time, how does it feel? And walking further forward into the future, looking out along the timeline and experiencing the struggle and dissatisfaction over all the years, how does it feel? Sometimes, you really need to stare the consequences in the face before you get the unconscious motivation to make the decisions and changes that you really want to make.

HOW ARE YOU MOTIVATED?

Meta-programs are the contentless strategies or processes by which we run our lives. We may be aware of the results of our meta-programs, but they are unconsciously run and maintained. However, if you understand your meta-programs, you can understand and manipulate what motivates you.

Madeleine is a sales manager of a team of eight. When times became tough and the team was struggling, Madeleine decided to 'motivate' the team by offering bonuses for higher sales. Two members actually got higher sales, but two remained unchanged and four actually got worse! What happened?

The answer to this puzzle is easy once you understand that each of us is motivated away from pain and towards pleasure. However, we are motivated in different proportions of 'towards' and 'away from' and individuals have a 'critical point' along a continuum that is their prime motivating point. The two members who improved were almost entirely 'towards' motivated, meaning that they were easily inspired

CHAPTER 12 YOUR SABOTAGING THINKING AND BEHAVIOUR

by the reward. The two members who remained unchanged actually needed to have a little 'pain' built in—without this, their motivation 'recipe' wasn't quite right. The four who got worse would possibly have improved if no bonus were offered, but instead the consequences of failure were made very clear!

Peter really wanted to eat more healthily. He had been successfully treating his food compulsions and addictions and now had a genuine desire to eat more fruit. He especially enjoyed icy-cold watermelon! His partner noticed a huge section of watermelon in the refrigerator and said, quite disdainfully, 'Who do you think is going to eat *that*! What a waste of money!'. Peter found he now couldn't eat the watermelon. Peter is almost entirely 'towards' motivated. Put a punishment or criticism in Peter's way and he will 'balk'. He doesn't do it deliberately and is upset that he can't simply 'ignore' what is for him a negative motivation.

How does this impact on you? Well, there are negatives and positives (pain or reward) attached to most things. There will be negatives and positives around being overweight, and negatives and positives around being slim.

If you are 'towards' motivated

If you are almost entirely 'towards' motivated, you need to eliminate all the negatives around being overweight and being slim, and remove all the positives around being overweight. In this way you are left only with positives about being slim. That is a 'critical recipe' for you, and provided you treat your food compulsions and so on, you are likely to remain slim once you reach this point. Keeping a 'slim' photo of yourself on your refrigerator door should work well!

If you are 'away from' motivated

If you are almost entirely 'away from' motivated, you need to build up and intensify the negatives about being overweight and make sure you eliminate all the positives about being overweight. Don't think about being slim at all, just focus on the pain of being overweight. There is a problem here for you once you reach 'slimness' because you may lose your awareness of the pain of being overweight that was such a powerful motivator for you. You might like to keep a few 'fat photos' around to remind you!

PART 3 SABOTAGE

If you are a mixture of 'away from' and 'towards' motivated

If you are a mixture of 'away from' and 'towards' motivated, you need to have at least some negatives still running associated with being overweight and some positives associated with being slim. You should ensure that you thoroughly eliminate all positives about being overweight and all negatives about being slim. You might like to keep a 'fat photo' around, but you should probably stay off the scales while you are going through the process. Use clothing size as an indicator instead.

An automatic, psycho-cybernetic propulsion system!

Once you've set up the motivation recipe that is just right for you, with the proper mix of 'away from' and 'towards' factors, you need to provide yourself with the driving force that ensures the system works automatically to propel you in the direction you wish to go.

Think of something that you do entirely effortlessly, almost without thinking. Is it a regular hobby? Brushing your teeth? Cooking dinner? The reason that this is so effortless and automatic for you is that it is state motivated. This means that there is an emotional state that comes into play whenever it is time for you to engage in this activity. You can think of it as a state of 'no alternative'. In other words, it would be unthinkable to do anything but this activity!

Are you getting an idea? Good! And yes, you will use the collapse anchors technique!

EXERCISE

You may want to read over the instructions for collapse anchors starting on page 32 before you attempt this exercise.

1. Get a sense of yourself being slim and healthy and intensify this feeling until you are coming *towards* the peak state. (Remember, if you wait until you're actually *at* the peak state, that's too late!) Quickly anchor this on your left knee and then break state by opening your eyes and concentrating on something neutral. Repeat this exact process twice more. From a neutral state, make sure you test this anchor to ensure that you have set it correctly.

106

CHAPTER 12 YOUR SABOTAGING THINKING AND BEHAVIOUR

2. Next, get the feeling that goes with your effortless activity and intensify this until you are coming into a peak state. Quickly anchor this on your right knee and then break state as before. Repeat this exact process twice more. From a neutral state, test this anchor as well.
3. When you are sure that both anchors are set, collapse anchors by first firing the 'slim' anchor and then two seconds later firing the 'effortless' anchor, saying to yourself as you do so 'And put that over the top of it'. Take off the 'slim' anchor first, followed two seconds later by the 'effortless' anchor and quickly break state. Repeat this exact process twice more.

Chapter 13
Using the meta model to stop criticism in its tracks: how not to get manipulated!

THE META MODEL is a model of language that demonstrates how language serves to limit and control you. When you become aware of the ways in which your own language, as well as the language of others, serves to imprison you, you are offered the keys to the prison gates!

This chapter will help you to:

✓ Use the meta model to identify the distortions, generalisations and deletions in your daily conversations.

✓ Use the meta model to form clever questions that spell death to distortions, generalisations and deletions.

CHAPTER 13 HOW NOT TO GET MANIPULATED!

The meta model

The meta model is a model of language that points out the language 'short cuts' we human beings use to communicate with each other and ourselves, and aids us in realising that our language can never represent the fullness of our experience. Whenever we attempt to describe our experience in words, we are exaggerating (distorting) actual experience, assuming patterns or similarity where they might not exist (generalising) or leaving things out (deleting).

When you understand the way that language violates 'reality', you have some pretty powerful ways to communicate, persuade and think logically instead of emotionally.

HOW CAN AN UNDERSTANDING OF THE META MODEL BENEFIT YOU?

When you understand the structure of language, you can challenge your own and others' communications so that you automatically understand that the world is much bigger than your conscious experience of it. In other words, challenging language violations literally 'melts' the illusions created by the distortions, generalisations and deletions that have been used.

The metal model teaches us to challenge language violations through an array of simple but highly effective questions. To use the meta model effectively, you must firstly learn to recognise language violations, and secondly learn to respond to these violations with particular types of questions.

Do the following exercise with a friend, cheat as much as possible and not only will you soon become an expert at recognising language violations, you'll also be able to deal with them very rapidly indeed!

Warning! If you attempt to debate or answer a person's claim, you are not using the meta model and all you are likely to get is a debate or an argument. Stick to questions only, with the view that you're merely seeking missing information!

PART 3 SABOTAGE

EXERCISE

1. Cut up some pieces of paper into 'flash cards' and write on each one the name of a meta model violation, as follows:

   - mind reading
   - lost performative
   - cause/effect
   - complex equivalence
   - pre-supposition
   - universal quantifiers
   - modal operator of necessity
   - modal operator of possibility
   - nominalisation
   - unspecified verb
   - simple deletion
   - lack of referential index
   - comparative deletion.

2. Sit opposite each other and hold up one card at a time. Your friend must make up a sentence that includes this particular meta model violation. In response, you have to ask a meta model question.

   For instance, you may hold up a card that says 'Mind reading'.

   Your friend might then say: *I know you want to make me a cup of coffee right now.*

   In response, you might say: *How, specifically, do you know I want to make you a cup of coffee right now?*

   Both of you can cheat as much as you like (by reading through the following descriptions of meta model violations)—the faster and more often you cheat, the faster you'll master the meta model!

To follow are some examples of meta model violations.

- **Distortions** bend the truth! Here are five types of distortions we all use:

  Mind reading (claiming knowledge of someone's internal state)

Example	*You don't understand me.*
Possible response	*How do you know I don't understand you?*

110

CHAPTER 13 HOW NOT TO GET MANIPULATED!

Example — *You don't want to lose weight.*
Possible response — *How, specifically, do you know that I don't want to lose weight?*

Lost performative (using value judgement)

Example — *Fatty food is bad.*
Possible responses — *Who says it's bad?*
According to whom?
How do you know it's bad?

Cause/effect (claiming that a 'self' is not at cause)

Example — *You make me upset.*
Possible responses — *How does what I'm doing cause you to choose to feel upset?*
How, specifically?

Complex equivalence (claiming that two experiences are one and the same)

Example — *Your taking time to exercise instead of spending it with me means you don't love me.*
Possible responses — *Have you ever lived a healthy life when you loved someone?*
How does my taking time to exercise mean I don't love you?

Pre-suppositions (using a statement that has to be taken for granted in order for a sentence to make sense)

Example — *If you knew how important this was, you wouldn't question my request.*
Possible responses — *How do you know I don't know?*
How am I questioning your request?

- **Generalisations** claim 'it's not just me, it's everyone'. Or they claim importance or even possibility or impossibility! Here are some examples:

  Universal quantifiers (claiming universality: all, every, never, etc.)

  Example — *You never stick at anything!*
  Possible responses — *Never?*
  What would happen if I did?

Modal operators of necessity (should, shouldn't, must, mustn't, etc.) and modal operators of possibility (can, can't, will, won't, etc.)

Example   *I have to be the one to do it.*
Possible response   *What would happen if you didn't?*

Example   *I can't take a day off.*
Possible responses *What would happen if you did?*
                    What prevents you?

- **Deletions** conveniently leave out information altogether! Here are some examples:

    Nominalisations (verbs that have been turned into nouns)

    Example   *Our communication leaves a lot to be desired.*
    Possible responses *Who's communicating what to whom?*
                        How would you like to communicate?

    Unspecified verbs (an incompletely described action)

    Example   *You're not trying.*
    Possible responses *How, specifically, am I not trying?*
                        Not trying what?

    Deletions (simple, lack of referential index or comparative)

    Example (simple)   *I am uncomfortable.*
    Possible response   *About what?*

    Example (lack of referential index)   *They say it's bad for you.*
    Possible response   *Who, specifically, says so?*

    Example (comparative deletion)   *He's better at it.*
    Possible responses *Better than whom?*
                        Compared to whom?

Once you've mastered the meta model, criticism by others becomes an incredibly amusing game! See the examples in the table below. Notice through all of these that I never ask 'why'. I ask how, where, when, what, in what way, who says, and so on, but I never ask 'why'. 'Why' doesn't fish missing information from a particular communication. Instead, it invites debate.

CHAPTER 13 HOW NOT TO GET MANIPULATED!

We're not interested in presenting logic, or in inviting debate or argument, we just want to 'rattle the slots' and expand the speaker's concept of reality, even if that speaker is us! And we can best 'rattle the slots' by finding the holes (every possible linguistic ambiguity we can identify or insert) in the critical statement.

Some of these response questions may seem rather silly to you. Imagine that you are the person making the statements. Read back the responses to yourself. How do you feel about the critical or limiting statements now? Perhaps the statements themselves seem *more* silly? Perhaps the person who made that statement would feel a little less attached to it now?

If you think this is fun, just wait until you learn 'sleight of mouth' when you do full NLP training! The meta model rattles the slots of criticism or manipulation, but sleight of mouth well and truly stops it in its tracks!

Some real-life examples you may have heard	Possible responses
Why don't you stop that silly diet for once and have some chips with me?	Do not say 'I'm not on a diet'. It doesn't work, and that's a refutation, not a meta model challenge. Try: *Silly in what way?* *Stop in what way, specifically?* *Diet?* *For once what?* *What silly diet?* *What would happen if I didn't?* *What chips?*
How can you say you're on a diet when you're eating cheese?	*Say in what way?* *Say how?* *When did I say I was on a diet?* *What diet?* *What cheese?* *How, specifically, did I say I was on a diet?* *What caused you to decide that I said I was on a diet?*

113

PART 3 SABOTAGE

Some real-life examples you may have heard	Possible responses
You don't look like you're losing weight to me.	*Look in what way?* *Losing in what way?* *Losing what weight?* *Who should I look like I'm losing weight to?* *Should I look like I'm losing weight to someone else?* *How would I look if I were losing weight?*
You should be at home to cook my dinner.	*At whose home?* *What dinner?* *Cook how?* *According to whom?* *What would happen if I didn't?* *What would happen if I did?*
You never do anything I ask.	*Never?* *What would happen if I did?* *Ask of whom?* *Do what?* *Anything?* *Nothing?*
No pain, no gain.	*Who says?* *According to whom?* *What would happen if there wasn't?* *What pain?* *What gain?* *Pain for whom?* *Gain for whom?*
You just don't listen!	*How, specifically, do you know that I don't listen?* *Listen to whom?* *Listen in what way?* *Never?* *Ever?* *What would happen if I did?*

CHAPTER 13 HOW NOT TO GET MANIPULATED!

Some real-life examples you may have heard	Possible responses
You're talking nonsense!	To whom am I talking nonsense? According to whom? Who says? What nonsense? Nonsensical in what way? How, specifically? What would happen if I didn't?
Good mothers put their children first.	Who says? According to whom? What good mothers? Put in what way? What children? What would happen if they didn't? First before what? And then? What prevents them?
This new diet will lose 10 kg a week!	What new diet? New in what way? Lose it where? Lose it for whom? Lose it in what way? Lose it how? Lose 10 kg of what? And then? Who says? According to whom? What would happen if it didn't? Which week?
You're looking drawn. Here, eat some chocolate cake!	Looking drawn to whom? Compared to whom? Looking drawn in what way? Who says? According to whom? Drawn how? What would happen if I didn't?

115

PART 3 SABOTAGE

Some real-life examples you may have heard	Possible responses
I just don't understand what's got into you!	*Understand?* *You don't understand in what way, specifically?* *Got into me in what way?* *What would happen if you did?* *What prevents you?*
I thought you didn't eat that type of food any more?	*You thought?* *Thought in what way?* *Didn't in what way?* *Eat in what way?* *Which type of food?* *What food?* *Any more what?* *How do you know that I don't eat that type of food?*
It looks like you're having a bit of a relapse.	*What looks like I'm having a bit of a relapse?* *To whom does it look?* *Looks in what way?* *How, specifically, do I look like I'm having a bit of a relapse?* *A bit?* *What sort of a bit?* *Having in what way?* *Relapse?* *According to whom?* *What would happen if I didn't?*
I thought you'd be at your ideal weight by now.	*How did you think I'd be at my ideal weight?* *Ideal?* *What ideal weight?* *And if I was?*
How long have you been doing this weight thing now?	*What do you mean how long?* *Doing what weight thing?* *Doing?*

CHAPTER 13 HOW NOT TO GET MANIPULATED!

Some real-life examples you may have heard	Possible responses
Shirley and Sharon are doing Jenny Craig and have lost loads of weight and look great!	Who says? Shirley who? Sharon who? According to whom? Doing what? Doing in what way? Who's Jenny Craig? Lost where? Lost in what way? Loads? Great in what way? What weight? And then? What would happen if they didn't?
You've tried this before. What makes you think it can work this time?	Tried in what way? Tried what before? Before when? Think what? What specifically makes you think that I think it can work this time? What can work this time? What do you mean 'work'? What time? What would happen if it didn't? What would happen if it did? According to whom? Who says?
If you give away those larger clothes, you're burning your bridges.	Give away to whom? Give away where? What larger clothes? Burning in what way? What bridges? Who says? According to whom? What would happen if I didn't?

117

PART 3 SABOTAGE

Some real-life examples you may have heard	Possible responses
This little dessert won't hurt. If you're so hung up about it, exercise more tomorrow.	Won't hurt in what way? According to whom? What would happen if it did? Hung up in what way? Hung up about what? How, specifically, do you know that I'm hung up? Exercise in what way? How much more? What would happen if I didn't?
I'm going to feel guilty eating this if you don't have some too.	How, specifically, have you chosen to feel guilty? Guilty in what way? Who says? According to whom? What would happen if you didn't? Eating what? Have what, too?
You have such amazing willpower. Do you think you can keep this up for the rest of your natural life?	How do you know I have amazing willpower? Who says? According to whom? What willpower? What would happen if I didn't? Keep what up? Natural life? What would happen if I didn't keep it up?
How much do you think you'll lose each week? What is your goal weight and when do you think you'll reach it?	How much what do I think I'll lose each week? (money, gambling bets, sheep?) What week? Lose in what way? What goal? Reach what? What would happen if I didn't?

CHAPTER 13 HOW NOT TO GET MANIPULATED!

Some real-life examples you may have heard	Possible responses
I'll put on my calendar that we can go for a pig-out to celebrate ...	Put on your calendar in what way? What calendar? What would happen if you didn't? Go where? What pig-out? Who can go for a pig-out? Pig-out in what way? Celebrate what? What would happen if we didn't?
Aren't you worried about losing muscle in addition to fat?	Worried in what way? What would happen if I weren't? Losing in what way? What muscle? What fat? What would happen if I did?
You don't want to go too far the other way and become anorexic.	How, specifically, do you know that I don't want to go too far? How far? Too far compared to what? Too far compared to whom? What other way? Anorexic? Anorexic in what way? What would happen if I did? What would happen if I didn't?

Make sure you attend to your own self-talk too!	Possible responses
When I'm slim, I'll be happy.	Who says? According to whom? When? Happy in what way? Slim in what way? What would happen if I weren't? What prevents me from being happy now?

Chapter 14
Putting your weight goals to the test

IT'S ONE THING to set a weight goal, but it's quite another to know with any certainty whether that goal is actually realistic or achievable. NLP wellformedness conditions constitute a 'litmus test' to help you to discover any loopholes in your goals.

This chapter will help you to:

✓ Check how realistic your goals are through the application of wellformedness conditions.

✓ Use the collapse anchors technique to ensure you reach your weight goal with ease.

CHAPTER 14 PUTTING YOUR WEIGHT GOALS TO THE TEST

Wellformedness conditions

NLP makes use of wellformedness as a way of checking how realistic and appropriate your goals are. Your weight goals should certainly be subjected to wellformedness conditions!

The term 'wellformedness' was first used in relation to the checking of therapeutic outcomes to see whether they were both realistic and ultimately desirable. This was done because sometimes what we think we want is not actually in our best interests, or even conflicts with other goals. Wellformedness conditions are now used as a goal-setting tool because the increased specificity and realism available through wellformedness enhances our ability to achieve our goal.

We know that when we are assessing a goal for its 'wellformedness' we are attempting to achieve both realism and 'fit'. We are doing our best to ensure that the goal is indeed not only achievable, but also that it is truly *desirable*. We are unlikely to be able to achieve or maintain a goal that is out of alignment with our own guiding principles or values.

To apply the principles of wellformedness, set out your weight goal using the following exercise.

Exercise

1. State your goal in the positive (not in the absence of a negative) and ensure you are talking about a physical goal, not an internal state or emotion.
2. Put your goal in context. How, where, when and why do you want this? Do not say 'in six months time'. Instead, nominate the date, for example 30 August 2004. 'Why' is incredibly important. If you do not have a sufficiently motivating 'why', you will not have the automatic 'energy' to achieve your goal.
3. Be sensory specific. Can you describe the achievement of your goal in all sensory representational systems? What will you see, hear, smell, taste and feel that will provide you with the undeniable evidence that you have achieved your goal? What sensory representational systems will inform others that you have achieved this goal? What will others see, hear, smell, taste and feel that will provide them with the undeniable evidence that you have achieved your goal?

PART 3 SABOTAGE

4. Make your goal self-fulfilled and self-maintained. Your goal must not rely on the contributions of others and it must not be subject to events outside your control. What resources do you have or must you acquire in order to achieve this goal?
5. Honestly evaluate the effects of achieving your goal. What will achieving the goal get for you? What will achieving the goal lose for you? What will not achieving the goal get for you? What will not achieving the goal lose for you? What will your goal cost you?
6. Ensure that your goal is in alignment with your other goals, values and guiding principles.

These are the classic NLP wellformedness conditions. I like to add one more:

7. Ask yourself whether you believe you can achieve your goal easily, safely and enjoyably. As you ask yourself this question, take special care to be aware of your physiological response. While you consciously may believe in the ease of achieving the goal, your unconscious mind may be coming up with all sorts of evidence for difficulty. If you get a low, 'flat' or other negative feeling in response to this question, follow the steps in the next exercise.

You can use the collapse anchors technique to ensure your unconscious mind interprets the goal as one that will be achieved quite easily.

Exercise: Making goals easy

1. On your left knee, install an anchor for 'achieving this goal'. (One woman who did this exercise used the thought of fitting into size 12 jeans 'straight off the rack'.) Really get into the feeling of achieving the goal and intensify that feeling until you are coming into a peak state. Quickly anchor this on your left knee and then break state by opening your eyes and concentrating on something neutral.
   Repeat this exact process twice more.

CHAPTER 14 PUTTING YOUR WEIGHT GOALS TO THE TEST

2. From a neutral state, test this anchor to ensure that it results in the same physiological response.
3. Now think of at least three instances where you achieved a goal with such ease that it seemed to happen by itself. If you haven't got these exact memories, don't worry—just nominate memories something like this.

    Are these memories powerful for you? Do they 'feel' really great to you when you relive them? If so, you can use them as is. If not, take some time now to 'ramp them up' by making a movie of how you would have liked things to happen and tell your unconscious mind to use that memory as if it really happened.
4. For each of these memories, install an anchor on your right knee (all in the same location). For each memory, really get into the feeling of 'achieving this goal with amazing ease' and intensify this feeling until you are coming into a peak state. Quickly anchor this on your right knee, break state as before and then repeat this exact process twice more.

    You now have a 'super-anchor' where three powerful examples of achievement are stacked together.
5. As before, from a neutral state, test this anchor to make sure that you've set it successfully.
6. Now think of your new goal, firing the 'achieving this goal' anchor as you do so. Then two seconds later fire the 'achieving this goal with amazing ease' anchor, saying to yourself as you do so 'And put that over the top of it'. As you feel that familiar sense of confusion or 'spaciness' say to yourself 'That's right' and release the 'achieving this goal' anchor first, followed two seconds later by the 'achieving this goal with amazing ease' anchor and then quickly break state. Repeat this exact process twice more.

You have just told your unconscious mind exactly what sort of ease you want to experience in achieving your new goal!

Chapter 15
Dealing with the impact of past failures

WE ARE VERY GOOD at reminding ourselves about how we have failed in the past. Often, we are so busy reminding ourselves of these failures that we practically live in the past! If you want to break free from the influence of your past, the NLP fast-rewind technique is one of the best ways to do so.

This chapter will help you to:

✓ Use the NLP fast-rewind technique to mess up your mental movies so that they entirely lose their impact.

CHAPTER 15 DEALING WITH PAST FAILURES

You're a movie mogul!

Many of us are so talented when it comes to running movies in our head (usually highly negative ones!) that we should have chosen a career as a movie director. Marie had a beauty. Whenever she thought about losing weight, in her mind she'd run over about three past failures, fast forward to 'now' and then watch herself failing to lose weight and continuing on to a catastrophic 'climax' where some disaster would happen (like her husband leaving her or being embarrassed being seen with her in public). She would fade out watching herself quietly weeping into a chocolate cake. She should have had a career in Hollywood!

One of the best ways I know to mess up a mental movie so that it entirely loses its impact is to use the NLP fast-rewind technique. When I tell you that I use this technique to wipe out the effects of trauma and torture for people with post-traumatic stress disorder, you'll understand that this is a technique that'll mess up your 'weight' movies just as well as it messes up some pretty scary movies for other people. If this technique can mess up something as severe as post-traumatic stress disorder, it'll make mincemeat of your weight movies!

The NLP fast-rewind technique

This interesting technique was first devised by one of the developers of neuro-linguistic programming, Dr Richard Bandler. Since then it has been improved upon by several practitioners and today the following version, described by Connirae and Steve Andreas in their most useful book *Heart of the Mind*, is probably the best known.

If you are running scenarios in your head, this is the perfect answer! To start the process, get a picture of a time just before a scenario starts to run, a time when all is well and you have no idea the scenario is about to start.

Warning! Do not start this exercise until you've read it all the way through and understand precisely what to do at each stage. If you don't follow the instructions *exactly*, it simply won't work.

PART 3 SABOTAGE

EXERCISE

1. Imagine that you are sitting in a movie theatre all by yourself, looking up at a blank screen. Onto the screen put a black and white still shot of yourself the day before the scenario commences—a time when you had no idea the scenario was about to run.
2. Float up from your chair into the projection booth at the back of the theatre. Notice that the window glass is very thick and that you are completely cut off from the theatre, although you can see and hear everything that is going on. Your focus should not be on the screen—instead, you simply should be observing yourself in the chair below and it is *this* self that is looking at the screen.
3. Run your scenario, starting from the still shot where you're comfortable and calm, progressing all the way through the scenario, and finishing well after the negative material is over and *everything has returned to normal*. This movie will take just a minute or two to run (i.e. it is *fast*). It is absolutely vital that you feel detached as the movie is playing. To do this, keep in mind that you are merely watching yourself watching the movie. If you feel any distress whatsoever, distance yourself further by imagining that you are going down to check on ticket sales or perhaps popping down to buy a hotdog while the movie comes to completion. Arrange for someone to 'come and get you' when the movie is over.
4. Let the movie run until the scenario is well and truly over and you are relaxed and comfortable again. Freeze the last frame of the movie and then float back down into your body in the chair below.
5. Get up from your chair and go up to the screen, jumping into this still frame (i.e. associate with the movie as if you are actually in it). Make the frame big, bright and colourful.
6. Run the movie backwards really fast so that it takes just seconds—like a rapid rewind. Feel yourself being pulled backwards through the movie in just seconds, all the way back to the beginning (the still frame of you at the start).

CHAPTER 15 DEALING WITH PAST FAILURES

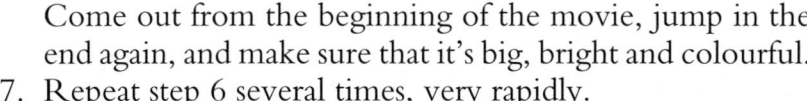

Come out from the beginning of the movie, jump in the end again, and make sure that it's big, bright and colourful.
7. Repeat step 6 several times, very rapidly.

The key to making this work is to remain dissociated throughout the process. That means no emotions at all! If you begin to feel any emotions, stop and dissociate, either by 'cutting yourself off' or by actually leaving the 'theatre' altogether. It may feel a little strange being pulled backwards at warp speed through your movie, but it should certainly not feel emotional.

PART 4
Food and exercise

Chapter 16
Ramping up your metabolic rate

Often, overweight people think that there is a problem with their metabolism. They are actually at least half-right!

This chapter will help you to:

✓ Understand what 'metabolism' really means.

✓ Discover eight ways to ramp up your metabolic rate and burn fat faster.

PART 4 FOOD AND EXERCISE

What is your metabolism?

The word 'metabolism' is used to refer to all the chemical processes that occur in the body to enable it to survive, grow and reproduce. You might also think of metabolism as the rate at which you convert food to energy (your metabolic rate). In fact, your metabolism is your very life force and, if it is low, you literally will feel as though the life has drained out of you.

Your metabolism is controlled by enzymes and hormones. Enzymes influence chemical conversations so that the necessary substances are made available as needed, and hormones control growth and the utilisation of chemical reserves.

Your metabolic rate may be fast or slow, or somewhere in between—in fact, each of us has an optimum level. Your metabolic rate is rarely a problem of itself, unless you were born with an enzyme deficiency. This means that if your metabolic rate is slow, it will rarely be because of some illness or genetic predisposition. Sorry, but these are the facts! If your metabolic rate is slow, there is a 99.99 per cent chance that it is slow because of your lifestyle!

BODY FAT SLOWS YOUR METABOLIC RATE!

Being overweight can lead to diabetes, thyroid and other hormone problems, and a slower metabolism, which in turn can lead you into a vicious cycle of being more overweight and having a slower metabolism. Very often, being overweight is the sole reason why someone suffers from depression!

The other way being overweight can dramatically lower your metabolic rate is that you don't feel like lugging all that fat around in order to do physical movement or take part in proper exercise. Without proper physical activity on a regular basis, many of the body's systems become sluggish, allowing the build-up of poisons in the body. In almost 100 per cent of cases, a slowed metabolic rate is due to inadequate or faulty nutrition and reduced physical movement!

Eight failsafe ways to increase your metabolic rate

Take heart—there are eight simple ways you can ramp up your metabolic rate. After years of abuse, it can take 6 to 12 months to get it going, but you can get it going!

CHAPTER 16 RAMPING UP YOUR METABOLIC RATE

1. EAT BREAKFAST!

If you don't eat breakfast, your metabolism will fail to kick in properly—in fact, it will never catch up, despite what you eat later in the day. Breakfast is essential to kick-start your metabolism and must properly provide what the body needs at that time of day. Deprive your body and your metabolism will slow down immediately.

Also, if you do not eat breakfast, the resulting drop in your blood sugar levels will have you screaming for high-energy foods by mid-morning. Your body will be so desperate for energy that it will create irresistible cravings for junk food that is high in fats or sugars. So breakfast kick-starts your metabolism and prevents mid-morning cravings. A double bonus!

And what are good breakfast foods? Certainly not simply toast and vegemite! For most people, high-fibre, unprocessed cereal is the perfect start (there are exceptions, so obviously other choices must be made by people who cannot tolerate cereals in their diets). Fruit is a great addition.

Also be sure to drink water. Some people say that they feel too nauseated to eat breakfast. This indicates a health problem and is not a normal, healthy response to waking in the morning. If this affects you, try taking just a couple of sips of water on wakening and see whether this makes a difference. If not, an orthomolecular review is required. An orthomolecular review will take account of your medical history and will examine the biochemical status of your blood and tissues. A doctor specialising in an orthomolecular approach will gain a deep understanding of your unique biochemical needs and what is required to bring you back to healthy functioning.

2. INCREASE YOUR WATER INTAKE

According to Dr Batmanghelidj, a world authority on the biochemistry of water, the majority of people in the world today are actually dehydrated. Many people mistake thirst for hunger and therefore eat instead of doing what their body really needs: drinking pure, clean water. Dr Batmanghelidj is in agreement with the famous Mayo Clinic regarding how to calculate the amount of water you require daily for optimum performance of all your body systems, including your metabolism. Simply divide your weight in kilos by 28. The answer is the number of litres of water you should be drinking on a daily basis.

3. DO SOME AEROBIC EXERCISE

It's sad that as we grow older we think in terms of 'exercise'. Remember when you used to call it 'play'? I hope after reading this that you will consider getting back some of that pleasure of moving fast, feeling the strength in your muscles, the wind blowing in your hair, and the oxygen coursing through your lungs and invigorating your whole body!

If you don't exercise, you end up with many problems, including a sluggish lymphatic system. Unlike your blood circulation system, your lymphatic system has no 'pump'—the only way the system gets activated is through muscle movement. That's why people who are confined to bed have problems with fluid build-up!

There are many, many health problems that occur as a result of letting our bodies stagnate—for example, circulation problems, an escalation of diabetes, cardiovascular disease, depression, an escalation of arthritic symptoms, and so on. Every health department in the world recognises this and the push is on to get people to be more active. Let's not kid ourselves that government departments are spending millions of dollars on advertising relating to physical activity because of any loving feelings towards us! They know that if people are more active, then literally billions of health dollars will be saved.

So how much exercise (I'm going to use the term 'play' from now on) do you need to do? Health professionals say that 30 minutes a day is enough to make a difference. But really, do you want to 'make a difference', or do you want to feel invigorated and alive?

To get the maximum benefit from your playtime, you need great aerobic activity for at least 45 minutes, at least three times a week. This doesn't mean you have to bust a gut at an aerobics class at the local gym. It simply means that for about 30 of those 45 minutes, you need to play at a level that allows you to comfortably hold a conversation, but puffing between the words.

Walking can do all of this very well indeed, and walking with buddies is a terrific way to start or end the day. Visit *www.walkingwithattitude.com* for exciting and inspiring walking information and challenges, including great tools to track your progress!

Swimming is a fabulous sport for strength, fitness, endurance, well-being and a host of other things, but it doesn't promote weight loss. The reason is that the coolness of the water both lowers metabolism and increases appetite! So do keep swimming, by all means, but add other land-based activities as well!

And remember, just because you're not a child anymore, it doesn't mean you don't have just as much right to go out and play! You wouldn't deprive a child, so don't deprive yourself of this essential part of life.

How many opportunities can you find to play now?

4. BUILD YOUR MUSCLES!

No, you don't have to look like Arnold Schwarzenegger in order to increase your metabolism. Many people are afraid to gain muscle because they worry that it will make them look even more bulky. This couldn't be further from the truth.

Muscle is far more dense than fat, so it takes up very little room compared with fat deposits. Also, because fat is not an organ and contains almost no blood vessels, it doesn't require energy to 'function'. Muscle, on the other hand, is a blood-rich organ that requires considerable energy to function. A healthy, well-muscled person probably uses about 5–7 times more energy simply sitting on a couch than an overweight person does walking! Also, overweight people often have very poor muscle structure, causing other health problems.

So building up your muscles will rapidly increase your metabolic rate! Great ways to do this include using weights and resistance bands, or even using a fitball (provided, of course, you've been shown how to use one correctly!). All that is required is 20 to 30 minutes, three times each week, and you'll be on your way to a feeling of strength and wellbeing, and an increased metabolic rate!

5. REDUCE STRESS

Stress can certainly reduce your metabolic rate. Depression/anxiety and a low metabolic rate go hand in hand. If you have mental health problems, you can probably assume that this will be playing havoc with your metabolic rate.

The science of psychoneuroimmunology is approximately 25 years old and shows categorically that your emotional state affects your health—not just your immune system, but practically every system in your body, including your metabolism.

PART 4 FOOD AND EXERCISE

If you're stressed, depressed, anxious or fearful, please seek help from an appropriately qualified and experienced person.

6. GET ENOUGH SLEEP

The sleep cycle is essential for the normal function of all body systems. This means that you should sleep soundly for some eight hours each night and wake in the morning feeling refreshed, remembering more than one dream but less than four. Too little or too much dreaming means a malfunction in rapid eye movement (REM) sleep, which is associated with dreaming. If your sleep cycle is disrupted, please seek help from an appropriately qualified and experienced person.

7. EAT WELL, GET LOTS OF VARIETY AND INCLUDE HEALTHY SNACKS

Eating well means having a nutritious breakfast, lunch and dinner. The more variety you enjoy, the more likely you'll be getting all the nutrients you need to run your body well. If you don't snack properly between meals, you'll almost certainly send your body into 'starvation' mode, reducing your blood sugar levels, creating cravings and lowering your metabolic rate.

8. BE CONSISTENT

All of the above will increase your metabolic rate, but only if you practise them consistently! These are the recipes for living well and it's up to you to use the techniques in this book to remove every single block you may have to utilising them in your daily life.

> ## CASE STUDY
>
> How Peter stuffed up his metabolism—and the solution!
>
> Peter came to me quite despondent. I had shown him how to successfully eliminate all his food cravings, as well as his non-hungry reasons for eating. I'd installed positive unconscious responses to thoughts about physical exercise. But Peter had a problem. He was eating healthy food, he was working out

CHAPTER 16 RAMPING UP YOUR METABOLIC RATE

with a personal trainer three times each week, walking, going to yoga and drinking plenty of water, but he wasn't losing weight. What could be wrong?

If Peter had been losing fat and building muscle, I would have been quite satisfied with no actual change in weight for up to a month (because the increasing weight of a little muscle could easily be much the same as the weight of a lot of lost fat). However, it was clear that Peter just wasn't building muscle mass from his workouts. After *three months* of solid training, he should have noticed some improvement, particularly in his upper body. This wasn't the case, and after initially dropping 3 kg, nothing more had happened. Peter felt extremely fatigued and depressed, and he wasn't sleeping well. With these symptoms, his metabolic rate had to be low, despite everything he was doing.

Realising something was amiss, I asked Peter to describe a typical day, including work and leisure routines and his menu. Peter's typical day was perfect except for two things: he had taken some poor advice about carbohydrates and fats and practically eliminated them altogether, *and* he was allowing himself to get into a really hungry state by skipping the important morning and afternoon snack.

Carbohydrates are absolutely essential for energy, both mental and physical. Without an adequate intake of carbohydrates, your body has little to burn when it exercises and so will burn muscle instead. Most of us eat too much carbohydrate, but Peter was seriously endangering his health by eating practically none. Fats not only provide important nutrients (e.g. the Omega 3s), but they also play many vital roles in body function, including regulating appetite! No wonder Peter suffered from a depressed mood and no energy and was failing to gain benefit from his workouts.

In addition, by allowing his body to remain unfuelled throughout the morning and afternoon, Peter actually moved into a 'starvation' state, resulting in a lowered metabolic rate!

The solution? I suggested that Peter immediately plan to eat a snack in the mornings and afternoons, such as fruit, yoghurt or cheese and biscuits. He also needed to add a little carbohydrate to his diet—a baked potato with lunch would do that. Additionally, he could add a delicious olive oil dressing to his evening salad.

With the right fuel, Peter's body can do the job it was designed to do and Peter will feel a whole lot better!

Chapter 17
Food: what's normal anyway?

MANY OF US EAT UNHEALTHILY and have forgotten what is normal! And how can we blame ourselves when we've been fed so much hype and misinformation about diet and nutrition?

This chapter will help you to:

✓ Learn what portion sizes are normal.
✓ Identify which foods it's normal to eat on a regular basis and which foods it's not normal to eat regularly.
✓ Discover ideas for healthy meals and snacks.
✓ Plan for success!
✓ Understand the big carbohydrate debate.

PART 4 FOOD AND EXERCISE

Portions are the key

Unless you enjoy counting kilojoules (and I absolutely recommend against it because it tends to make people obsessive about food!), the fastest way to gain an understanding of what is healthy is undoubtedly to look at portion management.

You can use the shape of your closed fist, or the palm, thumb and top joint of the thumb, as standard portion sizes, thus allowing you to forget all about measuring and counting. This way you can relax and just do portion management by 'feel'.

To follow are sample portions of various foods that are suitable for meals and snacks throughout the day. Keep in mind that these are in no way comprehensive, nor do they cater for special dietary requirements, which are beyond the scope of this book. Be certain to consult with your medical practitioner or qualified nutritionist if you are in any doubt whatsoever of the suitability of certain food types for your needs.

In addition, every day you should have:

- 1 or 2 servings of fruit
- at least 1 L water (preferably 2 L), with an extra glass for every non-water drink you have (e.g. tea/coffee, alcohol, juice, milk).

Breakfast

- 1½ fists of low-fat, no-sugar cereal, with ½ cup of skim milk and a serve of fruit
- A bowl of oatmeal and a slice of toast with tomato
- A slice or two of toast rubbed with garlic, a drizzle of olive oil, a smidgen of goats cheese, tomato slices and basil
- A small omelette and a piece of fruit
- A slice or two of wholegrain toast with vegemite and a boiled egg
- Toast with pate and a piece of fruit
- Egg and toast with some tomato on the side
- Toasted tuna and cheese, sprinkled with sprouts

Morning/afternoon tea

- 1 piece of fruit
- 1 Sao biscuit (or similar) with a very thin slice of cheese (no butter) or ricotta cheese (gherkins too!)

CHAPTER 17 FOOD: WHAT'S NORMAL ANYWAY?

- 3 non-fat crackers with 1 thumb-sized amount of cheese
- A small tub of yoghurt, no added sugar

Lunch and dinner

- 2 slices of wholemeal bread with salad
- 1 cup of soup (no cream—or just a small spoonful) with a very small bread roll
- 1 plate of salad greens, with a thumb tip of dressing, and a boiled egg
- 1 plate of salad greens, plus 1 palm-size piece of meat or fish
- 1 fist-sized portion of pasta, and a palm-sized portion of bolognaise or other accompaniment
- 6 small sushi rolls (may be dipped in soy sauce and/or wasabi)

FOODS THAT SHOULD BE EATEN RARELY

Many of us get into the habit of eating foods that contain enormous amounts of fats, flour and sugar on a daily basis as if that were normal. Here are some examples:

- pasta sauces
- pies, pasties and quiches
- battered or crumbed foods
- pizzas
- fried food
- baked dinners
- baked beans
- foods with cream (sauces or soups)
- mashed potato with butter and milk
- avocado
- cakes and biscuits
- nuts
- chocolate or other confectionery
- thickened casseroles or stews
- cheese (more than a thumb-sized portion).

If you find that you're eating these foods regularly, don't try to deliberately cut down! Use the collapse anchors technique until you no longer desire them. Remember, food deprivation causes food cravings!

In addition, consuming more than 1–2 glasses of wine or beer each day is too much. Likewise, every can of soft drink (even low-kilojoule) that you consume rapidly increases your risk of being overweight. It is important to treat your desire for soft drinks of any kind. If you do drink these items, make sure you drink at least the same amount of water immediately after having the glass of soft drink or the alcohol. Treat this until it becomes a habit.

Also keep in mind that while moderate consumption of alcohol has been linked with certain health advantages, no such link has been found with soft drinks! It is better to eliminate them altogether.

FOODS TO FALL IN LOVE WITH

Just as we often develop habits of eating foods that are highly damaging to us, we also develop a dislike of foods that are good for us. This is amazing, because these are the very foods that fill us with energy and a zest for life. These are the foods that allow our brains to function efficiently, so that we can think clearly and make decisions easily.

Perhaps people have come to associate these foods with dieting? It is not the foods that are the problem, but the diets!

Here are some foods to fall in love with!

FRUIT

If you can't yet eat fresh fruit (and don't worry if this is the case, because some fresh fruits are pretty tasteless due to early picking and artificial maturation), experiment with canned fruits with a little natural yoghurt. Make sure you get at least 1 serve of fruit each day (and preferably 5).

SALADS

When we think about salads we often think 'boring'. In my opinion, boring salads should be tossed out (if you'll pardon the pun!). Salads should be exciting! They should be so exciting that nothing else quite measures up! Try salads such as fancy lettuce salad (using different types of lettuce such as oakleaf, coral, cos and iceberg, and including both red and green leaves), Thai salad, mushroom and cabbage salad, and coleslaw. Add delicious herbs like fresh rocket, basil and tarragon, or even include something a bit spicy like a shredded red chilli. Make your own quick, easy and incredibly delicious dressings by whisking together balsamic or white wine vinegar with some quality olive oil.

CHAPTER 17 FOOD: WHAT'S NORMAL ANYWAY?

(For recipes, see *www.dietclub.com*. Of course, I'm totally opposed to the concept of dieting, but there are some really great recipes on the site!) In fact, you can use your imagination to make up exciting salads that are a delight to the eye, the mouth and the stomach! Once you've eaten salads like this, you'll want them in winter too!

What do you have with your salad?

I work pretty long hours and like most working wives I do a very unfair amount of cooking. So I really resent any meal that takes longer than 15 minutes to prepare and cook! You could call me the ultimate lazy cook!

Keeping it fast means keeping it simple. And keeping it simple also happens to mean keeping it healthy! So with salads you could simply add a can of tuna, or quickly grill a sausage, steak or chicken. If I've had the opportunity to bulk cook on the weekend and freeze portions of food, I might include a fist-sized piece of lasagne or some chicken with chorizo sausage and tomato.

What about vegetables?

Instead of salads, try vegetables like broccoli, or asparagus or snap peas, which cook in just seconds. I love to grab strange-looking vegetables from the supermarket because I love new tastes. Remember to eat red vegetables too: carrots, capsicum, sweet potato and pumpkin. Get as much variety in colour and flavour as you can.

To cook vegetables, try either steaming them or quickly stir-frying them—two great ways to do vegies fast!

One vegetable I don't have often in the evenings is potato. It's got nothing to do with kilojoules, because in fact potatoes don't have an excess of kilojoules. You might prefer to get most of your starchy carbohydrates earlier in the day too—you might find you'll sleep better and will also feel better in the morning.

What about pasta, rice and noodles?

These carbohydrates are just fine, but not what I regard as essential to health. They all feel pretty 'heavy' to me and I don't eat them much. If you're making a stir-fry, try rice noodles, which are a lot lighter on the stomach. If you're having enough bread and cereals, you probably don't need pasta, rice or noodles very often. When you do eat them, make sure they have plenty of flavour. For example, rather than plain steamed rice, it's so much nicer to fry some onion and garlic with the rice, and add some chicken stock and fenugreek for a quick 'pilaf' rice!

Do you need to learn about healthy cooking?

It's not uncommon to find that people have grown up in families where healthy food preparation is unknown. These people often feel very uncertain about what constitutes a nutritious meal and how to cook it. There are tremendous recipe books available now, full of exciting and tasty meals that are also extremely healthy and nutritious. In addition, there are wonderful free resources on the Internet—as noted above, check out *www.dietclub.com*.

Winter comfort eating

In winter, people often like to eat casseroles, soups, mashed potatoes and so on because of their warming qualities. There's absolutely no need to stop this just because you want to lose weight. Go ahead and enjoy these delicious foods, just treating any need you may have to eat more than you should. Generally, a fist-sized portion is absolutely plenty, and in particular soups are nutritious, warming and difficult to eat too much of! It's easy to treat desires or fears around portion management with the techniques in this book.

Planning

Even the best-laid intentions can run astray due to poor planning. To follow are some of the things you need to ask yourself in order to ensure that you have a supportive environment for the changes you are making.

- ❏ Have I made sure that good food is always available to me?
- ❏ Do I always have an attractive array of fruit at home and at work?
- ❏ Do I have fresh water available to me wherever I am?

CHAPTER 17 FOOD: WHAT'S NORMAL ANYWAY?

- ❑ Have I ensured that I get breaks at times when I need to fuel up my body?
- ❑ Have I made time available for play?
- ❑ Have I actually scheduled in time to work on my food and exercise issues?

If you plan, and if you use the techniques you've learned in this book to treat every single block to healthy eating and exercise habits, you will make changes that occur easily, naturally and permanently. And you will have a quality of life that you had previously only dreamed about.

THE CARBOHYDRATE DEBATE

Low-carb, high-carb, low-protein, high-protein, no fat, high fat, etc., etc., etc., ad infinitum!

If you're a baby boomer or older, you were probably brought up hearing just two things about food: 'Eat your greens' and 'Moderation is the key'. I guess there wasn't much commercial mileage in these sayings, particularly for the diet gurus, because since then we've been subjected to a barrage of unresearched, unscientific, unmitigated diet claptrap!

Experts go on and on about the 'obesity epidemic' and the problem of junk food, linking the two as if they had solid evidence of cause and effect. The fact is, most overweight people aren't overindulging on fast food (many do, but not 'most'). However, most overweight people *are* eating far too much starchy carbohydrate (high-glycaemic carbs).

Let me explain. Prior to the mid-1980s, carbs (including cereals and other grain products) were not high on the food pyramid. Overweight and obesity levels were nothing like they are today—*they were not rising, either!* Then the grain lobby started working on health departments the world over and, lo and behold, starchy carbohydrates were suddenly pushed on us as the food source we should most concentrate on if we want to be healthy. Suddenly, and I mean suddenly, overweight and obesity levels began to rocket skyward—and they have continued to accelerate since then.

In contrast, junk food consumption has risen steadily. There has been no corresponding jump in junk food consumption along with the jump in obesity rates. Put simply, although junk food is clearly not good for us, it is not to blame for our 'fat' epidemic.

PART 4 FOOD AND EXERCISE

So, what is to blame? Equally as clearly, the correlation is there between excessive starchy carbohydrate consumption, inactivity and weight problems.

DO *NOT* CUT OUT YOUR CARBS!

Do *not* cut out your carbs! I've put this in a heading because I know people tend to lean towards overkill (I'm guilty of that myself—I just love overkill!). Carbs are not bad, and cutting them out *completely* will not only slow down your metabolic rate, it will also make you sick! You absolutely need carbs! So, if you're a normal healthy person and your nutritionist advises you to cut out all carbs, run for the nearest qualified second opinion!

The question is, how much do you need? For the average person, the list below is perfectly adequate, and if all three are eaten fairly regularly on a daily basis, most people will be getting enough carbs.

- 1 bowl of good quality, unsweetened, unprocessed cereal
- 2–4 slices of good quality bread
- 1 small potato, or a fist-sized portion of cooked rice or pasta.

If you're small, obviously you need less. If you're a big, well-muscled person, obviously you need more. We each have different requirements.

If you're feeling tired, despite the fact that you exercise regularly, sleep well and manage your stress, then chances are you're not getting enough carbs.

Seek proper, expert advice on this. If someone starts advising you to go to extremes, insist they show you the properly validated scientific research to back it up. It is not enough to say that 'This is based on the XXX diet book' or whatever. Ask for the facts, not some fantasy fad.

Part 5
Planning to win

CHAPTER 18
Using a weekly food plan: shave up to 75 per cent from your shopping time and family food budget!

THERE'S NO DOUBT ABOUT IT: people who eat a wide variety of healthy foods are the healthiest, slimmest people on the planet. In your food plan, innovate, innovate, innovate! When you go shopping, deliberately seek out healthy foods you've never tried before, just for fun. After all, food should be fun, shouldn't it?

This chapter will help you to:
- ✓ Take advantage of a food plan or menu plan to save time and money.
- ✓ Use the 'triple dead-end sidewinder technique' to deal with any complaints about your cooking!

PART 5 PLANNING TO WIN

Do you hate shopping?

I hate shopping. In fact, I developed my method of planning and shopping for food not because I wanted to have a 'food plan', but because I hated shopping and knew that planning would dramatically cut down the time it took for me to go through the supermarket! I used to have competitions with myself to see how fast I could get the hell out of there! My record is just under 30 minutes for a full family shop for one week! I was really proud of this—boasted about it for the whole week to anyone who'd listen.

The major tip I can give you that will shave your shopping time in half is to spend 5 minutes over a cup of tea or coffee planning your menu for the week. My basic menu would look something like the one below. It's not stuck in concrete—I can change things around depending on how we feel at the time, but it's a great guide, it saves me thinking, and it sure cuts down my shopping and cooking time.

Saturday lunch	Fresh bread roll, sliced meat and salad
Saturday dinner	Grilled fish and salad
Sunday breakfast	Scrambled eggs on toast
Sunday lunch	Bread roll and whatever
Sunday dinner	Roast lamb, sweet potato, pumpkin, beans, with rockmelon (cantaloupe) for dessert
Monday dinner	Chicken sausages and salad
Tuesday dinner	Steak and salad
Wednesday dinner	Pork chops, mashed potato and peas
Thursday dinner	Spaghetti bolognaise and spinach
Friday dinner	Marinated chicken legs and salad

Once you have your basic menu, you can start to write your shopping list. Write in groups of items that are located together and in the sequence you walk through the supermarket so that you won't have to go back to a particular aisle. A sample pro forma based on my local supermarket is given below. I don't actually use a list with headings. I use any old scrap of paper that's nearest to hand and group things together roughly in the order I walk through the supermarket. I always

CHAPTER 18 USING A WEEKLY FOOD PLAN

go to the same store so I know exactly where things are and I don't waste precious time stuffing around looking for things.

Fruit & veg	Cleaning
	Kitchen supplies
Dog	Canned or bottled food/ condiments
Meat	
	Bread
Dairy & eggs	Pasta/rice

Make sure you list the ingredients for each of your meals, unless of course you know that you already have an item in your pantry or refrigerator. As well as your menu items, include the supplies you want to take to work—for example, fruit, cheese and crackers, lite yoghurts, bags of mixed salad, little cans of tuna, some sliced meat, and so on. If you keep this food in the refrigerator at work, it's a piece of cake to throw together a snack or lunch that is cheap, fresh, healthy and extremely fast! Also include things you need for the bathroom, kitchen and laundry, as well as any medical or hygiene supplies. This includes stuff like coffee, tea, milk and bread that are not menu items but that are required anyhow.

Important and amazing fact! Did you know that 75 per cent of a supermarket's income derives from impulse buying? This means that most likely 75 per cent of your shopping time and money has been an absolute waste. That's probably worth an extra family holiday every year!

Just think about it. When you went down to the shop to buy milk, what else did you come back with that wasn't on your mind when you went? You could have done without that, couldn't you!

So not only will a food plan encourage you to be healthier, it can save you up to 75 per cent of your family shopping bill!

There's a sample shopping list filled out according to my menu below (note that I haven't added the dog food, cleaning stuff, hygiene or personal items, pantry items that are already in stock or things I want to take to work for the week). You get the idea? Now is that easy or what! Just tick or cross off the items as you go around the supermarket and you'll be out of that store in no time! *And* you'll have saved precious time and money!

SAVE YOUR MENUS

Definitely save your menus. Once you've got quite a few, you should have a lot of variety available to you without having to constantly think up new menu plans. Just shuffle through them and choose one that appeals to you. Pop it on the refrigerator door using a magnet, and you and the whole family will be a whole lot better organised. Plus, your partner and children know what they're looking forward to!

MORE TIPS FOR CUTTING DOWN SHOPPING TIME

For starters, being organised in this way means that you won't have to shop through the week because you've forgotten things. It's a once-only shop. Fantastic! Here are some more great tips:

- Make sure that you eat before you go anywhere near the shop. Otherwise, not only will you buy things you really don't want, but you'll also tend to buy too much quantity. You might even feel exhausted or mentally foggy pushing the darn trolley around. Eat a good healthy breakfast or lunch before you go near the shop.
- Don't push the trolley up and down an aisle that contains only 1–4 items on your list. It's much faster to nestle your trolley into the head of the aisle or just into the aisle where it's not in anyone's way. Then you can quickly trot down the aisle collecting what you want and hightail it back to dump it in the trolley.

CHAPTER 18 USING A WEEKLY FOOD PLAN

Fruit & veg
Lettuce
Tomatoes
Cucumber
Mushrooms
Sprouts
Sweet potato
Potatoes
Pumpkin
Beans
Spinach
Rockmelon
Basil (fresh for spaghetti)
Onions

Dog

Meat
Chicken legs
Lamb for roast
Chicken sausages
Mince meat
Fish
Pork chops
Steak

Dairy & eggs
Eggs
Milk

Cleaning

Kitchen supplies

Canned or bottled food/condiments
Bottle of diced tomatoes
Tomato paste

Bread
Multigrain bread
Bread rolls

Pasta/rice

- Shop logically, avoiding double tracking like the plague: efficiency, efficiency, efficiency!
- Shop fast—within safety considerations of course. But don't dawdle. You mean business when you're in that place and your goal is to beat the clock and get back home so you can enjoy your time doing something other than shopping!

PART 5 PLANNING TO WIN

- When you get back home, make sure your family is trained to collect the bags from the car and put the shopping away. You've been the 'hunter'—now it's time for them to do their bit. After all, you're probably going to prepare the stuff for them: don't you think they should contribute *something*?
- Just one more tip. If, at the end of the week, your refrigerator still has quite a lot in it, you are buying way too much. If you've managed your shopping money well, if you've planned well, by the end of the week your refrigerator (not your pantry) should look like Old Mother Hubbard's cupboard!

What to do if you get complaints about your cooking

Well, straight off the bat, I don't think that one person in the family should have total responsibility for cooking anyway. Even if you're a housewife or a househusband, there's no way you're a house *slave*! If other members of the household work 9 to 5 or whatever, why should you be working 6 to 12? If the food is simple and the menu planned, there's no reason why others shouldn't take turns preparing the meals. Also, I like the rule that states 'Whoever prepares also cleans up'. That way, the cook doesn't leave the cleaner with an unholy mess!

If these types of meals are a change for your household, no doubt you'll get some whining and complaints. People will fight against what's good for them. So how do you deal with it?

Preparing the ground is an excellent idea. Generally, people don't enjoy sudden surprises—they respond a lot better when the situation is explained to them. People like it when they're given the *reason* for a change before the actual change is announced.

A fantastic NLP technique for dealing with potential complainers is the 'triple dead-end sidewinder' technique by Christopher Tomasulo. I just love it! Follow these steps:

1. Start by acknowledging or stating the problem.

    For example, if you feel your partner might have a problem with the changes you want to make to your cooking, you might say 'Darling, I'm really worried about our family's health'. Spell out exactly what you're worried about and why. Spend enough time to induce a feeling of agitation or concern in your listener. If

CHAPTER 18 USING A WEEKLY FOOD PLAN

they're not in this state, you've got more work to do so they really 'get' that there's a serious problem.
2. Suggest three rather poor solutions. In turn, demonstrate the futility or unpleasantness of each one. This is the 'triple dead-end' part. For example:

'We could stay just as we are. But with 65 per cent of all illnesses caused by exactly this sort of lifestyle, we'd be condemning ourselves and our kids to sickness. We all deserve better than that, don't we?'

'We could just completely cut out all the bad food and go on a really strict diet. But I've tried that before and I know it not only doesn't work, it just makes me cranky and hard to get on with. We don't want that, do we?'

'We could "make up" for our poor eating by cutting out alcohol completely. But I think it's nice sharing a wine over dinner, and anyway, a bit of alcohol is good for you, isn't it?'
3. Then fire the 'sidewinder'! Suggest the solution you want to put in place, demonstrating that it is much more preferable to the three dead ends you've already discussed. For example:

'Alternatively, darling, we could simply make a decision to concentrate on the sort of food that is tasty and really good for us. We'll all be a lot happier and healthier. We won't have to put up with useless, lousy diets. We can still enjoy having a nice wine together. And we'll have good fresh food, better and easier than before, giving us more time together as a family. I think we can even cut our food bill by up to 75 per cent! And we could use that for a nice holiday together, couldn't we?'

Chapter 19
Your weekly exercise plan

Over 90 per cent of people who take up an exercise program in order to lose weight regain their weight within 12 months. Why? Because they have failed to make physical activity a lifestyle change! This chapter provides an exercise plan that starts with where you are right now, and builds slowly and comfortably until you are at your optimum level for health and wellbeing!

This chapter will help you to:
- ✓ Appreciate the importance of choosing an enjoyable exercise routine.
- ✓ Start your exercise routine from where you are now.
- ✓ Identify normal aches and pains.
- ✓ Just do it!

CHAPTER 19 YOUR WEEKLY EXERCISE PLAN

This section is incredibly short, because it's really, really incredibly simple! In basic terms, if you want to be healthy and if you want to be slim, you **must** move your body. If you don't move your body enough, there's no doubt about it, sooner or later you will get mentally or physically sick, and you'll certainly die an awful lot sooner than you should—regardless of what you eat!

So, you can continue to do nothing or too little, but your health will just continue to slide, won't it? Or you can do some *boring* routine if you want, but how long do you think that will last? Or you can push yourself with a really *hard* routine, but you won't enjoy it and you won't keep it up, will you?

Alternatively, you can simply combine playing your favourite sport with a bit of resistance (weight) work. That way, you'll be 'getting out to play' rather than exercising, and you'll be rewarded by your weight work because stronger muscles let you play a whole lot better. Why do you think sports stars always, always, always do weight training as well? And you'd like to feel strong and gorgeous, wouldn't you?

Have you noticed what I just did? Did it stand out like the proverbial dog's hind leg? Yes! I used the triple dead-end sidewinder technique. And you can use it on yourself as well. Even when you *know* you're 'tricking' yourself, it will still work!

START BY DOING MORE THAN YOU DO RIGHT NOW

It's a huge mistake to suddenly go from being totally inactive to doing kickboxing training 10 times a week. You need to pace yourself for steady increases in activity until you're playing at a good level.

Right now, that might just mean walking around your house! Then you might walk around the block. Then you might move up to walking 3–4 km five or six times a week. Check out *www.walkingwithattitude.com* where you'll get lots of great advice and support for a walking routine. Get some buddies to join you and make it social and fun!

If you're taking up a sport, start small. If it's tennis, just play a set to begin with. If it's netball or basketball, keep subbing off every 5 minutes or so, until you can last the whole game fairly comfortably.

It doesn't matter *how much* you do, as long as you're doing *more*. The important thing is to always be pushing yourself just that little

PART 5 PLANNING TO WIN

bit. Once your routine becomes 'easy', you know it's time to step it up a little!

ACHES AND PAINS

It's quite normal to feel soreness when you first start exercising or playing. In fact, if you don't feel it, then your level of activity is ludicrously inadequate!

Check with your medical practitioner to see what starter level of activity is safe for you and what type of soreness is normal—and what might be a genuine sign that you're doing too much.

Just remember, your body is tough and resilient. It is meant to move, it is meant to be strongly challenged. It is actually designed and built that way. You are not a piece of fragile crystal, so go for it!

SCHEDULE IT IN!

Nothing happens without planning and exercise is no different. If you know you won't do it by yourself, coopt buddies to keep you on track. Once you've built up your strength and fitness, nothing will stop you! Check with your medical practitioner to make sure what you're about to do is appropriate for your health and wellbeing and *just do it!*

Slot in at least 3–6 sessions of sport or walking (cardio) activity each week. You *can* make time. Do it now, write it in your diary, display it on the refrigerator, tell the whole family—and *just do it!*

Slot in 3 sessions of strength building. This doesn't have to be tough. You can start with as few as 5 squats, sit-ups and push-ups, building up until you're doing 3 lots of 15–20 each. Or you can go to the gym 3 times a week or get a personal trainer. Do it any way you like, but *just do it!*

By starting small and building up, you'll ensure that you don't turn your play into 'punishment', that it's always an activity that pushes you and exhilarates you.

Concentrate on the great feeling of increased oxygen in your lungs and through your body. Take pleasure in observing how your muscles are becoming firm and strong. Notice how you are able to do more of the things you've been missing out on—with no effort at all!

If that's not quality of life, I don't know what is!

Chapter 20
One step at a time: using what you've learned in an effective manner

WHEN IT COMES TO MAKING CHANGES, many people gain a great deal of confidence if they have a good plan to follow. The last thing you want to do is to try to do everything 'overnight'—that's a fantasy that's destined to failure. Instead, let this plan take you, one step at a time, easily and naturally towards your weight goal.

This chapter will help you to:

✓ Understand what is meant by 'continuous' improvement—it's not always forward!

✓ Start from where you are now.

✓ Make small changes each week.

✓ Appreciate that it's not fast change that's important—it's real, permanent change!

PART 5 PLANNING TO WIN

A WEEKLY PLAN FOR CONTINUOUS IMPROVEMENT

When I say 'continuous' improvement, I'm not suggesting that all progress will be forward. That's not normal or natural. If you're doing it the right way, genuinely using the methods in this book to treat and eliminate every single negative unconscious response to food or exercise, you will notice improvements. You'll also notice 'backsliding' or even feelings of impatience, anger, disappointment, and so on. Just consider it all part of the process and keep treating! Share your experience with the WeightChoice chat list (see Appendix B for details how to join). You'll see that it's like this for most people.

Sure, you will probably find that this method takes longer to get results than does some crash or fad diet that you may have used in the past. The difference is, the changes you are making now are for good. You don't have to force yourself to go without. You're actually changing your food preferences. Remember, this is not a race. This is about your life. And you've got the rest of it to sort yourself out and make it better.

Many people will be quite happy to take it from here themselves, identifying and treating what they know is in the way for them. However, most people prefer to have a plan or strategy laid out for them—they feel safer that way. So, to follow is a week-by-week plan for getting on track and staying on track.

Some of you will fly through this 12-week plan in 12 weeks or even less. It depends on three things: (a) how much time you have to devote to self-treatment; (b) how much commitment you're willing to make to actually complete the treatment; and lastly (c) how complex or big your problems are. The more complex your problems, the longer it will take to work through them. Giving an extreme example, it's possible that someone could take 6 months to complete just 1 week of the plan that follows, and they might even need to call in expert help to complete one or more of the weeks. So treat this plan as a guide only, and do your best to stick to it, realising that it may take longer than suggested.

If you are able to stick to this plan, and genuinely achieve change not by willpower but through authentic change of unconscious preferences, then you will certainly have defeated everything that

CHAPTER 20 USING WHAT YOU'VE LEARNED

could possibly cause you to gain weight. You will be on track to gaining and maintaining your perfect, healthy weight and you'll never need to consider diets, kilojoule counting, tape measures or scales ever again!

WEEK 1

Before you start, re-read the section on NLP wellformedness in Chapter 14 (see pages 121–123). Write out a goal for your weight/health and run it through the wellformedness conditions.

Since it's more important to increase physical activity than it is to do anything else, it's logical to start with physical activity. In fact, you'll be considering physical activity every single week of the plan, because as soon as you find that your routine has become 'easy', you need to step it up!

This week, make a decision (if necessary with the help of your medical practitioner) about the level of physical activity that is best for you right now. Also arrange your schedule so that you have plenty of time to do this activity and absolutely commit to it.

Identify every single negative feeling (e.g. fear, resentment, dislike, anxiety, stress, embarrassment) you have about this activity and treat it. You can use EFT, BSFF, the resource triangle and anchoring. They all work really well. In fact, use the lot. Hit them with everything you've got until you absolutely love the feeling of the wind in your hair, the oxygen in your lungs, that gorgeous, sexy heat through your body and on your face, and that slippery wetness and aromatic freshness of a good sweat!

If you're out playing or exercising and you notice any negative feelings, treat them on the spot!

WEEK 2

How did you go with your exercise routine in Week 1? Was it too easy? If so, increase it a little. You might not have more time, but you can certainly add more effort—pick up the pace of your walking, stay on the tennis court 8 minutes instead of 5, or add weights to your squats or lunges. Push and challenge that gorgeous body—you will be shocked how much your body loves it!

Re-read the section on logical levels in Chapter 8 (see pages 60–62). Run through the exercise on pages 61–62, beginning at the environment level and imagining that you have achieved the goal you wrote about last week.

This week, concentrate on what you're putting into your mouth. It's a good idea to keep a food diary so that you can see exactly what you've been eating. A lot of overeating is done on automatic pilot and it can be quite surprising when you become conscious of what you've been doing. Just keep the diary and we'll check it out next week.

Week 3

Once again, check your exercise routine. Don't push yourself too fast, just make sure that whenever you notice it's easy you add a little bit extra. Not too much, just a little bit so that it's a bit more of a challenge for you. Just a little bit of soreness is generally perfect because it tells you your muscles are working as they should.

Now let's take a look at your food diary. Compare what you've eaten with the foods listed in the sections 'Foods that should be eaten rarely' and 'Foods to fall in love with' in Chapter 17 on pages 141–142. What changes, if any, do you need to make? Check your portion sizes against what is listed in the section 'Portions are the key' on pages 140–141. Are you in fact eating quantities that are too much for your body?

Write a list of the types of foods you should eat less of. Note down by how much your portion sizes need to decrease. Write down any negative feelings you have about making these types of changes (e.g. fear, resentment, anger, worry, stress, panic, sadness). Among these negative feelings, consider what this type of eating does for you. Does it mask unhappiness, loneliness or anger? Do you feel nurtured or even loved when you eat this food? Treat these feelings also. If you are using food as a crutch for real problems, you will have to resolve them right now. You may need to engage expert help to do this, but you deserve it!

This week, you should deal with all the negative feelings, not the food itself. Use any technique you like to eliminate these awful feelings forever. If you're in any doubt at all about *how* to do this, get onto The Lifeworks Group's WeightChoice chat list right away and ask the gang. They're there for you!

CHAPTER 20 USING WHAT YOU'VE LEARNED

Week 4

Check your exercise routine as usual. It's been nearly a month now since you started, and you should have substantially increased your level.

You may not have lost weight, but you might notice that your clothes are becoming a little loose. That's exactly what you should expect by now.

Re-read about BSFF in Chapter 8 (see pages 63–71). Ask a friend to muscle test you as you treat every self-esteem or confidence issue listed. Make a list of any negative thoughts you have about your weight or health and test for and treat these as well.

This week, deal with the food that you're eating but know isn't good for you. This might be chocolate, chips, pasta, pizza, bread, and so on. Whatever it is, this is the time to remove your addictive/compulsive feelings about these foods now and forever! Definitely use the collapse anchors technique. It is always successful.

Week 5

Check your exercise routine as usual, increasing intensity or duration as required. You should be noticing some rather nice muscle definition around now. Admire this in the mirror and congratulate yourself for being so gorgeous!

This week, look at your portion sizes. I used to put the same amount of food on my plate as I did on my husband's. I realise now it wasn't very bright, but it was a habit I got into (and there were some 'deservedness' issues running also).

What really worked well for me was to use EFT to tap on my thymus point (high on the sternum) as I was piling the food on my plate. I also used BSFF (just a quick command word aimed at the plate). Very, very quickly I found my arm stopping in mid air as I went to put on another load of food, together with a slight nauseous feeling in my stomach. I literally couldn't put it on the plate!

See whether you can almost eliminate carbs from your evening meal. Really, they're best eaten earlier in the day anyway. You don't need pasta or potatoes at night on a regular basis. Leave them out and pile up the salads and greens. You'll most likely sleep better and will feel a hell of a lot better in the morning as well!

Week 6

Check your exercise routine as usual, increasing intensity or duration as required.

If you're curious how you're doing, you might want to step on the scales. Scales aren't exactly the best measure (body mass index, or even clothing size, is far more relevant), but I just couldn't help myself. I'm a gloater by nature and I used to love gloating to myself whenever I noticed the tiniest of weight drops.

By the way, conversely, if you really hate the scales, it's a great idea to step on them and treat yourself with EFT. As long as you hate them, they rule you and that's not a good idea, is it? Similarly, if you get stressed or angry or whatever when you see clothes on a rack, or someone with a nice slim body, treat this too. It's all relevant—it's all tied up with your emotions around weight and identity.

So this week be really aware of any negative feelings you have around scales, tape measures, kilojoule counters, pictures of slim models, the sight of clothes that don't yet fit you, or friends and family members who are slimmer than you. Treat all these to eliminate those negative feelings once and for all!

Week 7

Check your exercise routine as usual, increasing intensity or duration as required.

This week, concentrate on adding pleasure to your activities, including eating good food and playing or exercising. To do this, re-read the section starting on page 32 on using the collapse anchors technique to add incredible pleasure and delight to food and exercise. Remember the 'yummy food noises' technique and use this too!

Week 8

Check your exercise routine as usual, increasing intensity or duration as required.

If you're doing it right, you should have lost 4–8 kg by now! If you have not lost this much weight, you need to get some expert help—now. The reason I say this is that it is crunch time for you now. You've admitted that there is something in the way of your acting in your

CHAPTER 20 USING WHAT YOU'VE LEARNED

own best interests. You need to find out what that is and treat it so that you stop sabotaging yourself. This can be tricky to do on your own and that's why I urge you to get help if you need it.

Now is the time to really identify things you might have been denying to yourself (like, for instance, having portion sizes that are still too big, or not snacking healthfully so that you end up overeating at meal times). Go ahead and treat these things now.

Alternatively, if you're quite sure that your eating and exercise habits are excellent, but you are still not losing weight, definitely speak to an expert to find out what's going on (this may be a nutritionist, a personal trainer or an orthomolecular specialist).

One of the things you should have noticed by now is an increased enjoyment of water. Most people need to drink about 2 L per day in order to be healthy, more if they're drinking tea, coffee or alcohol. And, of course, you'll drink more when you're exercising or playing!

My mother-in-law used to drink very little water. She lived on a few cups of black coffee a day and a milk drink with her dinner. It almost killed her. In fact, a couple of years ago we were called over to Sydney because she was 'dying'. She was in a foetal position and comatose, and doctors decided to put a subcutaneous drip in her tummy (just a few little drops of saline solution). Miraculously, she came back to life. Her whole body peeled, from head to toe, and she awoke and asked for orange juice. It turned out that she had become severely dehydrated!

So, never underestimate the importance of water. Drink at least 1 L per day, and if you have any resistance to this, *treat it*!

WEEK 9

Check your exercise routine as usual, increasing intensity or duration as required.

This week, look at how your family and friends are doing. It's time to really check in and see what changes they're experiencing, because when you see changes in them, you know for sure that the changes you are making are deep, authentic, lasting changes.

Consider how well (or not) you're dealing with these changes. Are you being firm but loving with your family? Are you spending more time with friends who are upbeat, happy, positive achievers? Are you being honest about your own reactions to family and friends and treating this? What more might you need to do?

PART 5 PLANNING TO WIN

WEEK 10

Check your exercise routine as usual, increasing intensity or duration as required.

This week, recheck your food habits. If you're eating junk food more than once every three weeks, eating more than a thumb-sized portion of cheese per day, nibbling on nut snacks, eating more than a fist-sized portion of rice/pasta per day or drinking more than two alcoholic drinks per day, then you have urgent treatment to do. Use the collapse anchors technique or EFT to address these issues. (I am not suggesting here that self-use of these techniques is adequate for the treatment of alcoholism! Alcoholism requires expert help from a psychologist or psychotherapist.) Re-read the list of foods that should only be eaten now and then in Chapter 17 and be completely honest with yourself.

Some of the things to consider in targeting your treatment are listed below. Consider these questions and treat them thoroughly.

- *Have I always made sure that good food is available to me?*
- *Do I always have an attractive array of fruit at home and at work?*
- *If I'm eating poorly, why am I overeating/eating poorly?*
- *What do I think/feel immediately before I overeat/eat poorly?*
- *What does eating do for me (what feelings/needs does it seem to fill)?*
- *How would I feel if this food or this quantity were denied to me?*
- *Do I think that I would be 'giving up' anything if I stopped eating in this way?*

WEEK 11

Check your exercise routine as usual, increasing intensity or duration as required.

When people learn archery and they're aiming to shoot the bullseye, they're not taught to aim *at* the bullseye. They're actually taught to aim *through* it to a point *behind* the bullseye. Goal setting is just like that. So, with your weight goal, what is the bigger goal *behind* it?

Also this week, think about your life. If you were to compartmentalise your life into eight segments, what would they be? You might come up with things like home and family, relationships, social, work, financial, spiritual, health and wellbeing, and emotional.

CHAPTER 20 USING WHAT YOU'VE LEARNED

Write down these eight headings and do a little daydreaming. Under each heading, write down your absolute ideal of how you'd like that part of your life to be. Point form is best. Next, take each point and put it through the wellformedness conditions. Then set a time frame, work out the steps and make it your goal to get every single one of them.

Consider how you might go about using the techniques you've learned in this book to eliminate every single block that stands in the way of achieving everything your heart desires.

WEEK 12

Congratulations, you're on 'maintenance'. If you were a dieter, you'd now be given a 'maintenance' diet that you'd be expected to stick to through sheer willpower for the rest of your life. But guess what? *No maintenance dieting allowed!* Yahoo! So what do I mean by 'maintenance'?

1. *I mean that you keep checking your exercise routine.*
   Whenever you notice that your exercise routine has become 'easy', just ramp it up a bit. You can do this in three ways:
   - Do it more often (more frequently, or, if it's weights, this might mean more repetitions).
   - Do it more intensely (faster walking or heavier weights).
   - Do it longer (e.g. play three sets of singles tennis instead of two).

   Now that's a recipe for incredible wellbeing, and a long and healthy life. You see those old guys belting around the tennis court at 80 and 90? I want to be just like them, don't you? That's a hell of a lot better than being some frail old soul in a nursing home!

2. *I mean that you keep checking your food.*
   From time to time you'll enjoy junk food and pigging out. No problem. Go ahead and enjoy it! You only need to pay attention if you notice it becoming a regular thing. If that happens, don't freak out, just treat it. Calmly and persistently treat it. It's perfectly normal, perfectly fine.

3. *I mean that you keep checking your emotions.*
   This means noticing whether you're experiencing inappropriate guilt or other negative feelings around food or exercise. Just keep a weather eye on your emotions and treat anything at all that comes up.

PART 5 PLANNING TO WIN

This is where true freedom lies! There's a whole new way of life out there, and if you keep on treating, you'll experience it for yourself.

Congratulations on reading and being part of this *sane* approach to weight and health. Not only are you assuring yourself of a wonderful, healthy life, your children, grandchildren and great-grandchildren will thank you for it!

APPENDIXES

Appendix A
Some medical reasons that may compound your weight problem: oestrogen dominance syndrome and copper toxicity

Medical problems relating to energy levels, cravings, depression or anxiety impact strongly on the digestion process and actually slow metabolism, particularly for women. If you are exercising daily and eating healthfully, yet are not moving towards a healthy weight, then it is essential that you undertake orthomolecular nutritional analysis (an examination of the biochemical status of blood and/or tissues) and rectify the complex biochemical chains that underpin good health and wellbeing.

Very few medical or health practitioners have the depth or breadth of understanding of biochemistry required to undertake such an investigation or to implement treatment. If this affects you, you need to find a qualified orthomolecular physician, and the best way to do this is to visit the web site *www.alternativementalhealth.com*, voted as the number one mental health site in the world and highly regarded by allopathic and complementary practitioners alike.

One range of symptoms for females that may alert them to the fact that biochemical issues are partially a cause of weight problems relates to oestrogen dominance. When oestrogen dominance is at play, a woman typically does not have enough vital elements and minerals to allow the proper take-up of zinc from her diet, resulting in many health problems, including the depression of progesterone and the build-up of copper from ovulation at mid-month. This syndrome is called oestrogen dominance syndrome, not because oestrogen is in excess, but because there is not enough progesterone in ratio to the oestrogen.

To make matters worse, if you have insufficient zinc in your body, your body doesn't tolerate the 'vacuum'. Instead, you absorb the next similar (two-valent) metal from the environment, and usually that metal is copper. Surprisingly, some copper is needed to function properly, but in this case too much is absorbed.

Once absorbed, the copper poses a real problem because it binds strongly to your tissues. It might not show up in blood samples (blood is so efficient at dumping what it doesn't need), but it certainly will show up in tissue samples. Typically, copper is laid down in the brain, liver and pancreas, creating a range of health problems. To make matters even worse, the copper produces a 'blocking' function to zinc, so you become even more depleted of this essential element.

Do any of these apply to you?

- depression
- headaches
- cravings
- dry or reddish skin
- water retention or bloating
- PMS/PMT
- gynaecological problems
- miscarriage
- cold hands/feet
- anxiety or even panic attacks
- memory or concentration problems
- sleep problems
- that 'hit by a truck' feeling first thing in the morning
- reduced libido
- gall bladder disease
- fatigue
- irritability
- hair loss.

If you have several of these symptoms and have made significant changes to your eating and exercise habits by using this book, but have not gained energy or lost weight, then it really is time to request full orthomolecular analysis of nutrition factors known to contribute to these and other health problems.

APPENDIX A OESTROGEN DOMINANCE AND COPPER TOXICITY

Simply taking zinc is not the answer, because the copper will fairly successfully block the take-up of zinc in your diet. Instead, an orthomolecular specialist will recommend a treatment called 'chelation therapy', which is usually a combination of herbs that have the chemical effect of binding with the copper, turning it into a form that can finally be readily excreted from the body.

Keep in mind that no chemical intervention, even natural intervention, will help solve a problem that is caused by the ongoing self-abuse of inadequate nutrition or exercise. If you continue to eat poorly or to avoid exercise, you are wasting your money.

In combination with a good eating plan, and a good exercise plan, intervention with chelation therapy can be literally miraculous.

Appendix B
Questions/troubleshooting

These questions and answers are taken from the WeightChoice chat list.

❓ Whenever I feel 'hopeless' (which can be quite often) or have been hurt by someone, I find treating an issue harder, because sometimes it just makes it worse. How do I get over this?

Sometimes, the apparent problem serves as a sort of decoy for deeper, more complex or more painful issues. This is one of the reasons I am so very much against untrained people 'doing therapy' with others. If you have a sense that the 'hopeless' feeling is in some way overwhelming, this is a sign that it's possibly not safe for you to proceed and that you need professional help from someone who can support you comfortably and safely through the process.

A lot could be happening here, but to follow are some suggestions:

1. When it 'gets worse', does it still feel like hopelessness or in fact has it now become fear, sadness or some other more distressing emotion? If so, it's not really the hopelessness that needs treating, but the emotion beneath it.
2. Consider in what way it 'gets worse'. Does this mean 'more painful' or is there indeed a sense of feeling overwhelmed by it? Often, when you feel overwhelmed it seems like there are many things going on, too many to deal with at one time. Chapter 5 provides step-by-step instructions for dealing with the feeling of being overwhelmed and should help you to get back to feeling comfortable quite quickly.

APPENDIX B QUESTIONS/TROUBLESHOOTING

3. The hopelessness may be quite complex of itself and may require persistence in order to get a satisfying result.
4. The particular treatment process you're using may not be the most appropriate. There are so many tools available that it isn't necessary to keep using one that isn't giving you the results you want. In fact, continuing to use an ineffective strategy, hoping to somehow get a different result the next time, is a good definition of insanity, isn't it?

> **I am trying to lose weight but am having trouble coming to terms with the fact that I don't need to diet. I'm feeling very unsafe not being on a diet!**

This is very understandable, especially for people who've spent most of their adult lives on diets! The feeling of being in a 'diet-free zone' is extremely unfamiliar! In addition, there can be a lack of trust at the level of the unconscious. Your conscious, logical mind can immediately appreciate the scientific facts that stack up against dieting. However, your unconscious mind doesn't operate on logic, it operates on automatic, conditioned learning. Remember when I talked about the unconscious mind being like an autopilot that's been programmed for a trip? If the programming is faulty, the plane will just keep flying, even if there's a mountain or storm ahead. The autopilot doesn't look around and decide for itself what to do. It just follows the 'rules'. And the feelings or emotions you have (like not feeling safe) are generated from your unconscious mind.

So you need to treat that programming and, of course, there are many ways to do this. If you were using the resource triangle, for instance (see Chapter 7), you'd need to decide on an appropriate trigger to think of while standing on the 'S'. This might be the thought of throwing out a diet book, the thought of getting fatter or anything else that brings up the 'not safe' feeling about abandoning dieting forever.

> **I fear that everything is going to be undone (as it has been in the past) so that I'll end up in a heap of self-sabotage, resulting in a panic attack!**

Wow! What a great movie you've been running! We often run these types of movies in our heads—sort of super-melodramatic catastrophe movies.

APPENDIXES

Perhaps you'd like to play around with a couple of things here? First, treat the fear of failure by taking those failure experiences from your past and treating each one individually. You'll probably need to treat 3–5 of them before the effect generalises across all of them.

Second, how about using the NLP 'fast-rewind' cure? This is a brilliant technique for messing up a lousy movie and it's fully explained in Chapter 15.

Finally, if you feel like having some fun, envisage a daydream that is just as extreme the other way—for example, deciding to lose weight and waking up the next day at your perfect weight, as if by magic. Rather than feeling self-sabotage and panic, you could build in some truly extreme narcissism where only the very best is good enough for you. See yourself turning your nose up at people, places and things that are in any way not in your perfect best interest.

> **Guilt is a huge issue for me. My guilt is with my sister (who looks fantastic by the way). She gets very down on herself, which gets me down because how could someone so beautiful feel so poorly about themselves? In order to identify with her, I find myself feeling guilty if I don't let her see that I feel as bad as she does. I'm one of those people that gets sympathy pains if someone close to me has a headache! I seem to take on everyone else's troubles.**

Guilt is a huge issue for many people, especially women. In fact, there's a whole section on this topic in Chapter 12. Much guilt can be treated using the resource triangle, EFT, BSFF (especially going through the process of addressing self-esteem issues) and even anchoring. You also need to treat any belief that you wouldn't be nice to people if you didn't feel for them. That's easy enough. In addition, a certain amount of behavioural modification is required because some of this guilt stuff definitely involves co-dependent behaviour. This is also discussed in Chapter 12, but I highly recommend that you read some books on co-dependence and further study the meta model. The meta model is a great way to prevent being manipulated!

> **Sometimes, pure embarrassment is enough to turn me into a puddle! For instance, I asked my husband if we should have dessert and his reply was a very condescending**

APPENDIX B QUESTIONS/TROUBLESHOOTING

'Okayyy'. This one word threw me into a very lonely pit in the bottom of my heart. Why should I react like this?

The way you've described embarrassment it's like an automatic reflex when you feel judged. And to you this means you then feel lonely and maybe quite sad. There is a lot of stuff happening all at once. This is great fodder for the resource triangle, which is perfect for treating 'chunks' of things. The 'S' could be your husband saying 'Okayyy'.

You could also use EFT, with your set-up sentence being 'Even though he said "Okayyy", deep down I know he really, really loves me' or 'Even though he said "Okayyy", I forgive him for being such a tactless pig'.

But where is the root of all this? Do you have childhood memories of being judged, embarrassed, isolated and sad? Each of these can also be treated. As usual, you'll probably need to treat three to five of them before the effect generalises across similar memories.

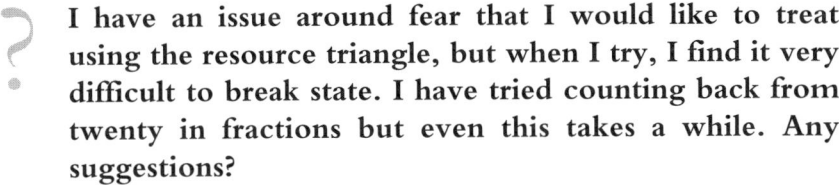 **I have an issue around fear that I would like to treat using the resource triangle, but when I try, I find it very difficult to break state. I have tried counting back from twenty in fractions but even this takes a while. Any suggestions?**

There are two reasons why it might be difficult to break state:

1. The issue is so contentious that you automatically get into the feeling of it too deeply. In this case, you might actually need someone to help you to come out of the state more quickly and cleanly. The resource triangle doesn't work well if you can't break state rapidly and cleanly. Alternatively, you could look at a photo that automatically gets you to a neutral state (e.g. a picture of a family pet or a picture of a tree) or perhaps you could rub your arm with an ice cube. If you can't break state, I'd suggest an alternative treatment method.

2. You are getting into the state too deeply. The 'S' requires you to merely get the trigger to the very beginning shred of the stuck feeling before leaping off and going neutral. It's not necessary to fully get the stuck feeling. In fact, this works against the method. You may have to think about the stuck feeling and decide where the very initial trigger is and just treat that.

177

APPENDIXES

> **❓ I find I am strongly resisting treating issues. What is the best way to treat this?**

This could be sabotage and might relate to self-image. If your unconscious mind has identity definitions that don't match your desire to lose weight, then certainly it will find ways to stop you. Alternatively, slimness may not 'fit' for your unconscious mind because of secondary gain issues relating to consequences of being slim or being overweight. It pays to keep treating self-image (and in my view BSFF is the very best way to do this) and to keep examining your gut reactions to thoughts of yourself being slim or being overweight. Your gut reactions are really your unconscious mind speaking to you.

Also, it could be that you're intending to treat yourself at times when frankly you are tired and really just need to chill out.

> **❓ What is the best method to stop snacking in front of the television? (Still doin' it!)**

It's not really a problem if you snack in front of the television as long as it's now and then and it's mostly stuff like fruit, for example. If you've successfully treated any desire for unhealthy food, you'll mostly choose the foods that are best for you.

This could also be a sign that you've been trying to control the snacking by willpower, thus creating resistance and a feeling of deprivation. Resistance is a sign that you haven't dealt with something sufficiently and have been trying to 'force' it.

Additionally, try getting some more insight into what could be happening for you. Sit in front of the television with a snack and say to yourself 'I'm going to put this back now' and see what feelings come up. This can help illuminate the real reason you have the desire to snack in front of the television.

> **❓ I have reached a plateau with my weight loss. Is this normal? How do I move on from here?**

It's normal to reach a plateau with your weight loss because you've actually reduced the amount of kilojoules you're eating. We now know, thanks to the work of nutritionist researcher Dr David Watts, that kilojoule reduction suppresses the stimulatory branch of the autonomic nervous system, thus working to reduce the metabolic rate. The body has to acclimatise to new eating preferences and this can take a little

APPENDIX B QUESTIONS/TROUBLESHOOTING

time. That's why it's so important not to go hopping on the scales—it's not your weight that's relevant, it's your habits and preferences that are the benchmark for your progress.

Of course, you have to be willing to consider and admit to things you may be doing that work against being a healthy weight. If you're not eating well, if you're not getting enough activity and if you're not doing the things that dyna-charge your metabolism, then you will reach a plateau that has nothing to do with your autonomic nervous system adjusting to a new way of living and everything to do with the fact that you're still not looking after your body.

If you're doing everything right, it's just a matter of time and you need to treat any feelings of impatience. On the other hand, if your weight remains at a plateau for over four weeks, it's time to check with both your personal trainer and your medical practitioner to determine what might be happening.

> **I've lost a few inches from my thighs and the skin is a bit wrinkly. Any good toning tips?**

This one's outside the ambit of the book but nevertheless very important! If you're dehydrated, then the skin can be wrinkly, but for toning tips the best person to talk to is a properly qualified personal trainer. Rapid weight loss doesn't give the skin a chance to recover very well and extremely obese people often require surgery to remove the excess skin. These people have to be very careful because they have little skin elasticity left. If they put their weight back on, they run the risk of splitting their poor overstretched skin. This is another reason why it's so important to avoid rapid weight-loss routines and instead focus on changing habits and preferences unconsciously.

> **If I eat something that's not good for me, I think I've ruined all the good I've done.**

Is this a conscious piece of logic, or is it a 'feeling' of having ruined all the 'good' you've done? If it's conscious, then it's something you can debate with yourself. You only have to look at all the cultures in the world that use ceremonial feasting and yet have no or few overweight people. You only have to think of all the slim people you know who occasionally eat chips, pizza, chocolate or whatever. Since you can only add 0.5 to 1 kg of fat in a week (constantly eating enough kilojoules to do so), it is literally impossible for you to 'ruin' anything by occasional pigging out or occasionally eating something that doesn't supply a terrific range of nutrients!

If it's a 'feeling', this means it's coming from your unconscious mind and definitely needs treating. EFT would be a great way to go about this—for example, 'Even though I've ruined all the good I've done, I choose to eat what I want when I want' or 'Even though I've ruined all the good I've done, deep down I know I'm worried about nothing'.

? How do I deal with the 'It's taking forever to reach my goal' feeling?

That fact that you've got this running means that you are impatient about reaching your goal. Anticipation, excitement and expectation are one thing, but impatience and struggle are altogether something else. This type of thinking means that you are conscious of not having your goal and is unhelpful because your mind tends to take you where you focus. EFT or the resource triangle would be a great way to attend to this issue. Also, if you are impatient, it can mean you don't like yourself as you are. The more you focus on your 'deficiencies', the more your 'deficiencies' remain. That's the nature of your mind: it takes you where you focus.

? What if the goal doesn't really seem in sight?

Even though a goal might be quite realistic and meets NLP well-formedness conditions, we know that some people will still have a feeling that it's not 'in sight'. For that reason, I've added a further condition to wellformedness that I think you'll find quite exciting! See Chapter 14 to learn why your mind needs examples of where you've succeeded with ease in the past and how to modify those examples and apply them to the goal.

? What should I do if I feel that I'm just dieting again?

You might feel this way because you're using willpower to deny yourself. If this is the case, you need to *stop*, because deprivation causes cravings and also impacts on your metabolic rate! However, if you've

APPENDIX B QUESTIONS/TROUBLESHOOTING

genuinely changed your tastes and preferences, then this feeling may be triggered by a similarity between what you are choosing now and what you chose when you dieted 'healthily' in the past. This needs to be treated again and EFT would be a great way—for example, 'Even though I feel like I'm dieting again (and maybe I'm just kidding myself), I choose to eat what I want when I want', and so on.

If you've found these questions and answers helpful, I urge you to join The Lifeworks Group's WeightChoice chat list. Just send an email to *info@lifeworks-group.com.au* and you'll be sent joining instructions. Once you've subscribed, you can send messages and get answers, as well as access the archives where there are more valuable questions and answers from previous discussions.

Appendix C
What now? Support, therapy

Support

There is very strong evidence that people who are isolated from others have difficulty losing weight. Even in the case of dieting (which I hope by now is well and truly a 'dirty' word for anyone reading this book), the programs that offer regular group support are the most successful. So, if you're serious about using the techniques in this book to achieve healthy, permanent weight management, you'll want to find a support group, or at least a group of friends who are keen to encourage and inspire each other.

Whether or not you are in a support group, you'll gain enormous benefit from joining a cyber support group. WeightChoice has a fully moderated group, run by staff fully trained in the WeightChoice approach, so you can relax in a safe and comfortable cyber environment without fear of flaming or spamming. To join, just email *info@lifeworks-group.com.au* and you'll be sent subscription instructions.

Therapy

The Lifeworks Group provides a therapy clinic in Perth, Western Australia, where people may be seen on a one-to-one basis. As at December 2003, the cost of a 50-minute session was A$178. (Contact The Lifeworks Group at PO Box 2018, Warwick 6020, email *info@lifeworks-group.com.au*, or visit the web site *www.lifeworks-group.com.au*.)

APPENDIX C WHAT NOW?

For elsewhere in Australia, or throughout the world, go to *www.energypsych.org*, the official site of the Association for Comprehensive Energy Psychology (ACEP), an international peak body for the new psychotherapies. It is not generally recommended that enquirers use other web sites for the simple reason that very many unqualified or untrained people are listed there. The field is not well regulated and is in relative infancy, so charlatans abound. At this stage, it is very much 'buyer beware' and you should thoroughly check the credentials of anyone professing to be a 'therapist' to ensure that they have at least minimum qualifications as a counsellor or psychologist.

Useful terms

addiction a physical or psychological need for a substance.
aerobic exercise exercise that demands increased oxygenation. Examples include brisk walking, jogging and kickboxing.
anchoring an NLP term used to describe the creation of an association between some sensory stimulation and an inner state (e.g. a certain song makes you feel a certain way every time you hear it).
Be Set Free Fast (BSFF) a psychological technique developed by Dr Larry Phillip Nims. It enables people to engage the unconscious mind strategically and systematically to make changes that achieve physical and mental wellbeing.
BMI see *body mass index*.
body mass index (BMI) a statistical measure calculated by comparing height to weight. A range of 20 to 25 is considered to be healthy, but individuals with well-developed muscles will discover that the BMI is next to useless. Using BMI measures, Brad Pitt is considered to be overweight, while Sylvester Stallone is obese! Why? Muscles weigh much more than fat!
BSFF see *Be Set Free Fast*.
carbohydrate chemically, a carbohydrate is any compound consisting of carbon and water. The best carbohydrates have a low glycaemic index, which means that they are less readily absorbed and converted to blood sugar. Almost all foods contain carbohydrate, but we need to eat fewer high glycaemic index carbohydrates (e.g. cakes, hot chips, white rice and pasta) and more low glycaemic index carbohydrates (e.g. fruits and vegetables, wholegrain pasta and legumes).

USEFUL TERMS

collapse anchors an NLP technique that can be used in a variety of ways to eliminate or enhance emotional responses. It can be used as an 'aversion' technique to beat addiction or as an 'attraction' technique to become enamoured of exercise.

compulsion the perception that you are 'forced' to engage in a behaviour.

conditioned response an automatic, unconscious emotional or physical reaction that occurs spontaneously with a particular stimulus.

diet merry-go-round a term used to encapsulate the uselessness of kilojoule-restricted dieting to achieve any sort of permanent change.

ecology when we talk about the 'ecology' of a problem or issue, it means all the social/psychological/spiritual/mental/physical components, not just of the problem itself, but of overlapping or connected problems. As in natural ecology, in our own inner ecology, no problem exists in isolation, but in fact affects every part of the 'system' in some way.

EFT see *Emotional Freedom Techniques*.

emotional eating eating not as a result of appropriate hunger, but in order to help cope with emotions.

Emotional Freedom Techniques (EFT) a neuro-somatic technique developed by Gary Craig that enables us in most cases to very rapidly eliminate negative or distressing emotional states.

food triggers/anchors stimuli that result in conditioned responses relating to food and eating behaviours.

GaugeWork an NLP technique developed by Astra Johnston. It makes use of the mind's capacity to achieve change through metaphors.

ideal body weight a weight range that is accepted as being healthy for a particular individual; it varies between countries.

kilojoule-restricted diet any diet or eating plan that is based on using willpower to eat a diet that contains reduced kilojoules (or energy) in order to lose weight.

kinaesthetic anchor an anchor is an association between some sensory stimulation and an inner state. A kinaesthetic anchor uses touch to induce a certain state.

logical levels see *neurological levels*.

lymphatic system the body's natural drainage system, which allows excess fluid to be eliminated from the tissues, at the same time flushing toxins and other matter from the body.

metabolism the process of chemical change in the body.
meta model a model of language and a structure for eliciting missing information, including the deletions, distortions and generalisations that make up common speech/thought.
modelling initially from NLP, a variety of techniques that allow us to take on the abilities or characteristics of others.
muscle testing isolating and challenging a muscle in order to determine the relative strength of muscle lock in response to a particular thought.
neuro-linguistic programming (NLP) a vast field incorporating human perception, language, cognition, performance and behaviour. Understanding the principles and tools of NLP allows us considerable personal power to run our own brain and creatively determine our own reality.
neurological levels originally from a branch of linguistics, and later developed in NLP, a way of categorising a hierarchy of consciousness.
neuro-somatic therapy any therapy that involves stimulation of the nervous system by simultaneously impacting on the body (touch, light, sound, etc.) and on brain function.
neuro-somatics a relatively new field, possibly a subset of NLP, which incorporates systematic stimulation of the autonomic nervous system to collapse or extinguish unhelpful conditioned responses to a very wide range of stimuli.
NLP see *neuro-linguistic programming*.
obesity being 20 per cent or more above the ideal body weight.
oestrogen dominance syndrome a condition whereby the ratio of oestrogen to progesterone favours oestrogen after the midpoint of the menstrual cycle. Often results in toxic deposits of copper and problems with gynaecological, digestive, thyroid and a number of other functions.
overweight being more 10 per cent or more above the ideal body weight.
overwhelmed a feeling of being emotionally overcome by the enormity or complexity of a problem or problems.
psycho-cybernetic system a sequence of unconscious processing that is self-generated and maintained.
resistance exercise exercise that challenges and builds muscle (e.g. weightlifting, fitball and resistance bands).

USEFUL TERMS

resource triangle an NLP technique developed by American master trainer Rex Steven Sikes that helps break down conditioned responses and rapidly eliminates the ability of people or events to cause us distress.

subconscious mind see *unconscious mind*. These terms are used interchangeably. If the world's leading lights in psychiatry and neurology cannot agree what it should be called, or even if it exists, I'm certainly not going to get fussed about it!

timeline therapy an NLP concept originally developed by Steve Andreas, and later commercialised and popularised by Tad James.

unconscious mind see *subconscious mind*. That part of our thinking process that is beyond conscious awareness.

WeightChoice an individually structured program, trademarked to The Lifeworks Group, which involves identifying eating, exercise and metabolic factors that have led to unhealthy weight gain, and systematically eliminating these factors at the level of the unconscious mind so that the person makes changes not from willpower or determination, but because preferences have changed genuinely and permanently.

wellformedness conditions a set of conditions from NLP, used to test the reality and realism of a goal.

BIBLIOGRAPHY

American Heart Association (2001), *Circulation: Lack of Scientific Evidence for High-Protein Weight-Loss Programs*.
Andreas, C & Andreas, S (1989), *Heart of the Mind*, Real People Press, Utah.
Bandler, R & Grinder, J (1975), *The Structure of Magic: A Book About Language and Therapy*, Science and Behaviour Books, Palo Alto, CA.
Bandler, R (1996), *Time for a Change*, Meta Publications, Capitola, CA.
Commonwealth Government Department of Health & Aged Care (2001), *Promoting Healthy Weight*, Commonwealth of Australia.
de Vernejoul, P et al. (1985), 'Etude des Meridians d'Acupuncture par les Traceurs Radioactifs', *Bulletin of the Academy of National Medicine* (Paris), 169, pp. 1071–5.
'Dieting Daughters Influenced by Parents' (1999), The Body Conference, sponsored by the Victorian State Government, July.
Egger, G (1998), 'Obesity and Weight Loss', Radio National.
Gallo, F (1999), *Energy Psychology: Explorations at the Interface of Energy, Cognition, Behaviour and Health*, CRC Press, Boca Raton, Florida, Chapter 1, pp. 10–15 and Chapter 3, pp. 33–49.
Health, V & Kausman, R (date unknown), *The Great Dieting Myths Dispelled*, International No Diet Day Literature.
James, T (1988), *Timeline Therapy and the Basis of Personality*, Meta Publications, Capitola, CA.
Life Tools for Success! (a monthly electronic journal supporting weight management and other quality-of-life changes), The Lifeworks Group, Perth.
National Health and Medical Research Council (1997), *Acting on Australia's Weight: A Strategic Plan for the Prevention of Overweight and Obesity*, Commonwealth of Australia.
Nims, L P (1998), *Be Set Free Fast Training Manual: A Dynamic System for Eliminating Distress and Creating a Fulfilling Life*, 2nd edition, published by author, Orange, CA.

BIBLIOGRAPHY

NSW Health Department (2000), 'Why 1500 Women a Year are Dieting to Death', *Sydney Morning Herald*, February.
Rand, A (1976), *The Fountainhead*, Signet.
Rossi, E L (1986), *The Psycho-Biology of Mind-Body Healing: New Concepts of Therapeutic Hypnosis*, Norton, New York.
Satir, V (1988), *The New Peoplemaking*, Science & Behaviour Books, Mountain View, CA.
Sell Your Way to Your Dreams: A Revolutionary Approach to Selling and to Life, The Lifeworks Group, Perth.
Sutherland, C (1999a), *Unlimited Confidence & Charisma! Fast Track to Personal Power*, The Lifeworks Group, Perth.
Sutherland, C (1999b), *Unlimited Freedom: Stop the Things That Stop You!*, The Lifeworks Group, Perth.
Sutherland, C (2000a), *Neuro-Somatic Treatment for Depression: A Preliminary Report on a Group Treatment Program*, The Lifeworks Group, Perth.
Sutherland, C (2000b), *The Lifeworks Joy Inventory: A Positive Instrument for Measuring Depression*, The Lifeworks Group, Perth.
Sutherland, C (2001a), *A Neuro-Somatic Approach to Treatment of Chronic Unresolved Physical Pain*, The Lifeworks Group, Perth.
Sutherland, C (2001b), *A Neuro-Somatic/Neuro-Linguistic Approach to Improve Behavioural and Academic Performance*, The Lifeworks Group, Perth.
Sutherland, C (2001c), *NLP in 10 Days: A Step-By-Step Training Program*, The Lifeworks Group, Perth.
Sutherland, C (2004), *You Don't Have to Accept Chronic Pain: Beyond the TENS Machine!*, The Lifeworks Group, Perth (forthcoming).
Tabrizian, I (2002), *Nutritional Medicine: Fact and Fiction*, 4th edition, NRS Publishing, Perth.
University of Western Australia & WA Health Department (1999), *Physical Activity Levels of Western Australian Adults*.
WA Health Department (1998), *Health Risk Factors, Private Health Insurance, and Health Service Data*.
Watts, D (1993), *Weight Control Through Metabolic Control*, Interclinical Laboratories, Gladesville, NSW.
Watts, D (1999), *Trace Elements and Other Essential Nutrients: Clinical Application of Tissue Mineral Analysis*, Trace Elements, Writer's B-L-O-C-K, Addison, Tex.
Wolpe, J (1958), *Psychotherapy by Reciprocal Inhibition*, Stanford University Press, Stanford, p. 668.
World Health Organisation (1981), *Global Strategy for Health for All by the Year 2000*, WHO, Geneva.

Index

Page numbers in **bold** print refer to main entries

aches and pains, **158**, 162
acupuncture, 76, 78
addiction, x, **28–9**, 30, 163, 184
aerobic exercise, 43–4, **134–5**, 184
afternoon tea, **140–1**
alcohol, 19, 142, 165, 166
'algorithms', 77
amygdala, 10, 78
anchors and anchoring, **31–2, 33–6**, 37–8, **44–6**, 52, 53, 107, 122–3, 161, 184 *see also* collapse anchors technique
anger, 4, 5, 19, 49
anxiety, 135, 136, 171, 172
Ashtunga Yoga, 44
Association for Comprehensive Energy Psychology, 183
attitudes
   exercise &, **40–7**, 57
   unhelpful, **20–1**
auditory anchors, **31**, **39**
automatic 'failsafe' system, 11
automatic thinking/behaviour, xi, 49
autonomic nervous system, 6, 75, 78, 178, 179
autopilot, **59–71**
'away from' motivation, 104, **105–6**

Bandler, Richard, xi, 26, 125
Bateson, Gregory, 60
Batmanghelidj, Dr, 133

Be Set Free Fast, xi, **xii**, 16, **63**, **65–71**, 92, 98, 100, 161, 162, 176, 178, 184
beach walking, 44
'Beat cravings, shift fat!' workshops, **28–32**
behaviour level (logical level), 60, 61–2
behavioural modification, 176
behavioural strategies, 73
belief(s), **20–1**, 57, 63, 64, 89, 98, **99–100**
beliefs and values level (logical level), 60, 62
beverages, 19, 142
   see also alcohol; water
biochemical issues, **171–2**
blob, the, **41–2**
blood sugar, 133, 136
body awareness, **46–7**
body fat, 6, **41–2**, 46, **132**, 135, 137
body mass index, **184**
boredom, 49
brain, 6, **9–11**, 49, 78, 142, 172
bread, 146
breakfast, 21, **133**, 136, **140**
breathing exercises, 47
BSFF *see* Be Set Free Fast

caffeinated beverages, 19, 165
Callahan, Dr Roger, **77**, 78
capabilities level (logical level), 60, 62
carbohydrates, **137**, 138, 143, **145–6**, 163, **184**
carbonated beverages, 19, 142
cause/effect, 111

INDEX

cereal, 140, 146
change consequences, **98–102**
change techniques, **23–94**
cheese, 141, 166
'chelation therapy', 173
chicken leg fantasy, **55**
childhood, **14**, 177
children, ix, 4, 7, 90
Chinese medicine, 76, 78
chocolate, 27, **28–9**, 32, **34–6**, **50**, 141, 163, 179
circuit training, 44
coffee and tea, 165
collapse anchors technique, **32–6**, 37, **38–9**, **44–6**, 106, 107, 122, 141, 163, 164, 166, 185
collarbone points, 81, 82
comfort eating, 6, 30, 49, 51, **144**
command word, **65–6**, 67, 68
commitment, 58, 160
communications, 109
complex equivalence, 111
compulsion, x, 29, 185
conditioned response, 10, **14–15**, 78, 185
conscious mind, 9, 11, 175, 179
consistency, 136
continuous improvement weekly plan, **160–8**
cooking, **144**, **154–5**
copper, 171, 172, 173
Craig, Gary, xii, 78
cravings, 8, 19, 25, 30, 32, 136, 141, 171, 172, 180
crown point, 82
cycling, 44

daydreaming, 167, 176
deaths, 4, 8, 41, 43
decision-making, 10
dehydration, 133, 165, 179
deletions, 109, **112**
depression, 21, 42, 49, 52, 132, 135, 136, 137, 171, 172
deprivation, ix, xii, 4, 8, 25, 141, 178, 180
diet merry-go-round, **4–6**, 185
diet problems, **7–8**
dietary fat, 19, **137**
dieting, ix, **4–8**, 182
  see also kilojoule-restricted diet
digestion, 171
Dilts, Robert, 60

dinner, **141**
disgust, 19, **35–6**
distortions, 109, **110–12**

eating disorders, ix, 4, 7
eating triggers *see* food triggers/anchors
ecology, **185**
'ecstatic' anchor, 46
EFT *see* Emotional Freedom Techniques
embarrassment, **176–7**
emotional eating, 22, 185
Emotional Freedom Techniques, xi, **xii**, 16, **75–87**, 161, 163, 164, 166, 176, 177, 180, 181, 185
emotional overwhelming, **86–7**, 186
emotional responses, 10, **18–21**, **48–58**, 167
  see also negative feelings/thoughts
empowerment, 26–7
energy, xii, 20, 21, **76**, 78, 171
environment level (logical level), 60, 61, 62
enzymes, 132
Ericksonian language, 52
example deletions, 112
exercise
  aches and pains from, **158**, 162
  anchoring &, **44–6**
  attitude to, **40–7**, **57**
  body awareness &, **46–7**
  emotions and behaviours involving, **20–1**
  focus on, **42–4**
  maintenance of, **167**
  metabolic rate &, **134–5**
  scheduling of, **158**
  starting your, **157–8**
  types of, **43–4**
  weekly plan for, **156–8**, **161–2**, 163, 164, 165, 166
  see also aerobic exercise
eyebrow point, 82

failure, x, **124–7**, 137, 176
family, **100–1**, 165
fantastical thinking, **99–100**
fast food *see* junk food
fast-rewind technique, **125–7**, 176
fasting, 6
fat (body), 6, **41–2**, 46, **132**, 135, 137
fat (dietary), 19, **137**

191

INDEX

fatigue, 21, 49, 137, 172
fears, 20, 21, 35, 49, 137, 176, **177**
   see also phobias
feelings *see* emotional responses; negative feelings/thoughts; positive thinking
fitball, 43, 44, 47, 135
fluid build-up, 134, 172
food
   examples to be eaten often, **142–3**
   examples to be eaten rarely, **141–2**
   metabolic rate &, **133**, **136**, 137–8
   planning, **144–55**
   see also breakfast; cooking; healthy food; junk food; menus; snacks
food addiction, x, **28–9**, 30, 163
food behaviours, **18–19**
food cravings, 8, 19, 25, 30, 32, 136, 141, 171, 172, 180
food deprivation *see* deprivation
food diary, 162
food emotions, **18–19**
food habits, 14, 22, 27, **166**
food plans, weekly, **149–55**
food portions, 19, **140–1**, 163, 165
food rewards, 14, 18, 49
food thoughts, 18, 19
food triggers/anchors, 19, 22, **25–39**, **48–58**, 185
free weights, 44
friends, **101**, 165
frontal cortex, 10
fruit, 133, 137, 140, **142**, 144, 178

Gauge Work, **89–93**, 185
generalisations, 109, **111–12**
Grinder, John, xi, 26
guilt, 5, 14, 18, 20, 27, 57, **102**, **176**
gustatory anchors, **31**
gym, 44

habits, 14, 22, 27, **166**
health problems, 3, 4, 7, 8, **41**, **42**, 43, 132, 134, 135, **171–3**
healthy food, 19, **36–9**
hippocampus, 10
hockey, 44
hopelessness, **174–5**
hormones, 132
hypnotherapy, 11

ideal body weight, 89, 185

identity level (logical level), 60, 62
ideomotor responses, **63–4**
impulse buying, 151–2
internal resistance, 90
internal settings, **88–94**

junk food, 133, 145, 166, 167
K27s *see* collarbone points
karate chop point, 80
kickboxing, 44
kilojoule-restricted diet, 6, **7**, 185
kilojoules, 143, 178
kinaesthetic anchors, **31**, **32–6**, **37–9**, 185

language, **108–19**
language patterns, 52, 55, 78, 79, **80**
language violations, **109–12**
learning, 10
libido, 6, 7, 172
lifestyle, **14–16**, 29, 132
The Lifeworks Group, xi, 13, 27, 162, 181, **182–3**
logical levels *see* neurological levels
loneliness, 49
lost performative language violations, 111
lower lip point, 82
lunch, **141**
lymphatic system, 42, 134, 185

maintenance, **167–8**
medical problems *see* health problems
memory, 10, 42, 87, 123, 172
men, 4
mental movies, **125–7**, 175–6
mental pictures, 9, 91
   see also Gauge Work
menus, **150**, **152**
meridian lines/points, **76**, 77
meta model, 52, 102, 104, **108–19**, 176, 186
metabolic rate, 5, 6, 7, **21–2**, 42, **131–8**, 171, 178, 180
metabolism, **132**, 179, 186
metaphors, 91, 98
Milton Model, 52
mind reading, 110–11
mind-sets, 101
modal operators of necessity, 112
modelling, 26, **73–4**, 186
morning tea, **140–1**
motivation installation, **102–7**

INDEX

movies *see* mental movies
muscle, 41, 42, 46, 162, 163
muscle building, **135**, 137
muscle locks, 64
muscle testing, **63–5**, **66–7**, 68, 69, **98–9**, 163, 186
muscle wasting, 21

National Nutrition Survey, 4
negative feelings/thoughts, 21, 51, 53, 56, **75–87**, 161, **162**, 163, 164
neuro-linguistic programming, 11, 13, 16, 29, 78, 100, 113
  background to, xi–xii, 26–7
  definition of, xi–xii, 26–7, 186
  fast re-wind technique &, 125–7, 176
  modelling techniques &, 26, 73–4, 186
  resource triangle technique &, xi, 51–8, 102, 161, 176, 177, 180, 187
  timeline technique of, 52, 102–7, 187
  'triple dead-end sidewinder' technique &, 154–5, 157
  wellformedness conditions &, 121–2, 161, 180, 187
  see also anchors and anchoring; collapse anchors technique
neurological levels, **60–2**, 186
neuro-somatic therapy, 75, 186
neuro-somatics, xi–xii, 186
Nims, Dr Larry Phillip, xii, 63
NLP *see* neuro-linguistic programming
nominalisations, 112
non-hungry eating, 48–58
noodles, 143–4
nutrition, 8, 136, 137–8
nuts, 141, 166

obesity, ix, 3, 4, 8, 145, 179, 186
  see also overweight
occipital ridge point, 82
oestrogen dominance syndrome, **171–2**, 186
olfactory anchors, **31**
orthomolecular review, 133, 171, 173
outer eye point, 82
overeating, 5, 28
  see also food portions; pigging out
overweight, **3–8**, 13, 41, 98, 132, 145, 186
overwhelmed feeling, **86–7**, 186
oxygen, 42

pasta, 143, 146, 163, 166
Pavlov, I., 14–15
perception, 49
phobias, 52, 77, 79, 93
physical movement *see* exercise
pigging out, 18, 167, 180
pilates, 44
play *see* exercise
pleasure principles, **36–9**
positive thinking, x, 58
precision (anchor setting), **33**
pre-suppositions, 111
problem behaviour, **17–22**
progesterone, 171
psycho-cybernetic system, 186
psychoneuroimmunology, 135
pump exercises, 44

Qi Gong, 47
questions, **174–81**

Rand, Ayn, 77–8
REM sleep, 136
resistance, **178**
resistance bands, 43–4, 47, 135
resistance exercise, 157, 186
'resource state', 52, **54**, **55**
resource triangle, xi, **51–8**, 102, 161, 176, 177, 180, 187
resting metabolic rate, 21
reward, 14, 18, 49
rice, 143, 146, 166
rollerblading, 44
rubbing points, **81**

sabotage, 14, **21**, 30, **95–128**, 165, 176, 178
safety issue, 98
salads, 19, **142–3**, 163
Satir, Virginia, 100
secret eating, 18, 27
self-care, 102
self-confidence, 68, **69–71**
self-esteem, xii, 68, 163
self image, **59–71**, 178
self-talk, **119**
sensory systems, **31**, 35, 53
shopping, **150–4**
skin wrinkles, **179**
sleep, 21, **136**
sleep problems, 42, 137, 172

193

INDEX

'sleight of mouth', 113
snacks
  healthy, 21, 136, 137, 165, **178**
  unhealthy, 18, **50–1**, 166, 178
social eating, 19
soft drinks, 19, 142
sore spot, 81
soups, 144
spirituality/purpose level (logical level), 60, 62
'spoiling' sessions, 47
sport(s), **43**, 44, 47, 57, 134–5, 157, 158
squash, 44
stair/step climbing, 44
starchy carbohydrates, **145**
starvation, 6, 136, 137
state management, 52
stimulus–response process, 10, 11, **15**
strength building, 158
stress, 18, 21, 27, 49, 51
stress reduction, **135–6**
subconscious mind, 9, 10, 11, **12–16**, 22, 27, 32, 53, 55, **63**, 64, **65–8**, 69, **89–93**, 102, 122, 123, 175, 178, 180, 187
support, **182**
swimming, **43**, 134–5

tapping points, 77, 78, **79–84**, 163
tea and coffee, 165
techniques, **23–94**
television, 18, 27, 49, 52, **57–8**, **178**
tennis, 43, 44
thalamus, 10
therapy, **182–3**
thinking *see* mental movies; negative feelings/thoughts; positive thinking
thought field therapy, **77**
thymus point, 80, 163
timeline technique, 52, **102–7**, 187
tiredness *see* fatigue
Tomasulo, Christopher, 154
top lip point, 82
touch football, 44
'towards motivation', 104, **105**, **106**
transformational grammarians, 26
treadmill, 44
triggers to eating, 19, 22, **25–39**, **48–58**, 177
'triple dead-end sidewinder' technique, **154–5**, 157

troubleshooting, **174–81**

unconscious conditioning, **14–15**, 25
unconscious mind, 9, 10, 11, **12–16**, 22, 27, 32, 53, 55, **63**, 64, **65–8**, 69, **89–93**, 102, 122, 123, 175, 178, 180, 187
unconscious programming, **12–16**
under eye point, 82
underarm point, 80, 82
universal quantifiers, 111
unspecified verbs, 112
unworthiness, 102
'uproar' game, 100

value judgements, 111
values, 89
vegetables, **143**
Vernejoul, Pierre de, 76
visual anchors, **31**
vomiting, 19

walking, 20, **43**, **44**, 47, 134, 135, 157, 158, 161
water, 21, **133**, 140, **165**
water retention, 134, 172
Watts, Dr David, 6, 178
weekly continuous improvement plan, **160–8**
weekly exercise plan, **156–8**, **161–2**, 163, 164, 165, 166
weekly food plans, **149–55**
weighing scales, **164**
weight disorders, 13
  see also obesity; overweight
weight goals, **120–3**, **180**
weight loss plateau, 178–9
weight training, 44, 135, 157
WeightChoice, 160, 162, 181, 182, 187
wellformedness conditions, 121, 161, 180, 187
willpower, x, 4, 14, 27, 43, 58, 118, 178, 180
women, 4, 7, 19, 171–2, 176
wrinkly skin, 179

Yogacise, 44
yummy noise factor, 39, 164

zinc, 171–2, 173